P9-AEU-445

POCKET GUIDE TO

GOOD
FOOD

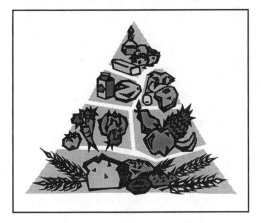

MARGARET M. WITTENBERG

✻

The Crossing Press • Freedom, CA 95019

ACKNOWLEDGMENTS

Much love and thanks to....

Everyone at The Crossing Press, especially Dennis Hayes and Elaine Gill for their much valued support and encouragement.

My husband, Terry, and our four-legged "children," Mochi, Betty, Scooter, Kitten Marie, and Junior, for giving me the space and understanding I needed while writing this book.

© Copyright 1996 by Margaret M. Wittenberg
Cover Illustration by Mike Monteiro
Cover Design by Sheryl Karas and Victoria May
Book Design by Sheryl Karas
Printed in the U.S.A.

Cautionary Note: The nutritional information, recipes, and instructions contained within this book are in no way intended as a substitute for medical counseling. Please do not attempt self-treatment of a medical problem without consulting a qualified health practitioner.

The author and The Crossing Press expressly disclaim any and all liability for any claims, damages, losses, judgments, expenses, costs, and liabilities of any kind or injuries resulting from any products offered in this book by participating companies and their employees or agents. Nor does the inclusion of any resource group or company listed within this book constitute an endorsement or guarantee of quality by the author or The Crossing Press.

ISBN 0-89594-747-1

CONTENTS

The Pocket Guide to Good Food is designed as a handy reference guide for you to take along with you wherever you go grocery shopping—in a natural foods store, food co-op, conventional supermarket, gourmet specialty food store, or even a farmer's market.

Using the Food Guide Pyramid as a basic organizational guide, each section of the book provides at-a-glance information about what to look for when shopping for the most nutritious, best-tasting, high-quality foods, including how much to buy, how to store them for optimum nutrition and safety and how much time they take to prepare. You'll also find a glossary of key terms that relate to the specific food groups, as well as a list of additives to avoid when reading labels.

For more information about the various foods and nutritional concepts and how they fit into an optimum diet, pick up a copy of *Good Food: The Complete Guide to Eating Well*, the comprehensive food and nutrition resource that details much more in depth what this pocket shopping guide merely hints in passing.

Enjoy!

—Margaret Moothart Wittenberg

HOW TO PLAN GOOD FOOD MENUS

THE FOOD GUIDE PYRAMID

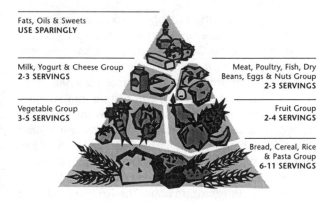

Fats, Oils & Sweets
USE SPARINGLY

Milk, Yogurt & Cheese Group
2-3 SERVINGS

Meat, Poultry, Fish, Dry
Beans, Eggs & Nuts Group
2-3 SERVINGS

Vegetable Group
3-5 SERVINGS

Fruit Group
2-4 SERVINGS

Bread, Cereal, Rice
& Pasta Group
6-11 SERVINGS

HOW MANY CALORIES DO YOU NEED?

activity level	calories/pound
inactive	12
lightly active	15
moderately active	16-20
very active	21-25
extremely active	25-30

THE NEW FOOD LABEL AT A GLANCE

Serving sizes are now more consistent across product lines, stated in both household and metric measures, and reflect the amounts people actually eat

The list of nutrients covers those most important to the health of today's consumers, most of whom need to worry about getting too much of certain items (fat, for example), rather than too few vitamins or minerals, as in the past

The label will now tell the number of calories per gram of fat, carbohydrates, and protein.

New title signals that the label contains the newly required information.

Calories from fat are now shown on the label to help consumers meet dietary guidelines that recommend people get no more than 30% of their calories from fat.

% Daily Value shows how a food fits into the overall daily diet.

Some daily values are maximums, as with fat (65 grams or less); others are minimums, as with carbohydrates (300 grams or more). The daily values are based on a diet of 2000 and 2500 calories.

Nutrition Facts

Serving Size 1 cup (255 g)
Servings Per Container

Amount Per Serving

Calories 70   Calories from Fat 15

	% Daily Value*
Total Fat 2g	**3%**
Saturated Fat 0g	**0%**
Cholesterol 0mg	**0%**
Sodium 250mg	**10%**
Total Carbohydrate 13g	**4%**
Dietary Fiber 3g	**14%**
Sugars 4g	
Protein 3g	

Vitamin A 70%	•	Vitamin C 20%
Calcium 4%	•	Iron 10%

* Percent Daily Values are based on a 2,000 calorie diet. Your daily values may be higher or lower based on your calorie needs:

	Calories:	2,000	2,500
Total Fat	Less than	65 g	80 g
Sat Fat	Less than	20 g	25 g
Cholesterol	Less than	300 mg	300 mg
Sodium	Less than	2,400 mg	2,400 mg
Total Carbohydrate		300 g	375 g
Dietary Fiber		25 g	30 g

Calories per gram:
Fat 9 • Carbohydrate 4 • Protein 4

SERVING COMPARISONS BY CALORIE LEVELS

Food Group	Sedentary women some older adults children (about 1600 calories)	Sedentary men moderately active women, teen girls (about 2200 calories)
Bread Group	6 servings	9 servings
Veg. Group	3 servings	4 servings
Fruit Group	2 servings	3 servings
Protein Group*	2-3 servings	2-3 servings
Milk Group**	2-3 servings	2-3 servings
Total Fat (20%)	36 grams	49 grams
*** (30%)	53 grams	73 grams
Total Added Sugars****	24 grams or 6 teaspoons	32 grams or 8 teaspoons

*1 serving protein=2-3 oz. meat, fish, poultry, tempeh, tofu or 1 cup beans or 2 eggs.

**Women who are pregnant or breastfeeding, teenagers, and young adults to age 24 need 3 servings of milk or an appropriate substitute for calcium.

***Showing both 20% calories from fat as well as the 1990 US Dietary Guidelines maximum of 30% fat, an amount which is generally considered too high. One gram of fat equals 9 calories.

Teen boys active men active women (about 2800 calories)	Very active men & women (3400 calories)	Extremely active men & women (4000 calories)
11 servings	13 servings	15 servings
5 servings	6 servings	7 servings
4 servings	5 servings	6 servings
3 servings	3-4 servings	4 servings
2-3 servings	3 servings	3 servings
62 grams	75 grams	88 grams
93 grams	113 grams	133 grams
44 grams or 11 teaspoons	52 grams or 13 teaspoons	60 grams 15 teaspoons

****Using a maximum of 6% of total calories allotted to added sugars. Added sugars include those which are deliberately added to sweeten or foods/beverages which are primarily simple sugars such as soft drinks. It does not include naturally occurring simple carbohydrates in foods as found in fruits, dairy products, grains, and beans. One teaspoon equals 4 grams of sugar.

NUTRITION FACTS LABEL: NUTRIENT NEEDS FOR DIFFERENT CALORIE LEVELS

Total % Daily Value for each of the nutrients listed on Nutrition Facts label (Fat*, Saturated Fat, Total Carbohydrates, and Dietary Fiber) can add up to:

TOTAL CALORIES	FAT (20%)	FAT (30%)	SATURATED FAT	CHOLESTEROL
1600 calories	55%	<80%	<80%	<100%
2000 calories	68%	<100%	<100%	<100%
2200 calories	75%	<110%	<110%	<100%
2500 calories	84%	<125%	<125%	<100%
2800 calories	95%	<140%	<140%	<100%
3400 calories	115%	<170%	<170%	<100%
4000 calories	135%	<200%	<200%	<100%

TOTAL CALORIES	SODIUM	TOTAL CARBS	FIBER
1600 calories	<100%	80%	80%
2000 calories	<100%	100%	100%
2200 calories	<100%	110%	110%
2500 calories	<100%	125%	125%
2800 calories	<100%	140%	140%
3400 calories	<100%	170%	170%
4000 calories	<100%	200%	200%

*Percentage values for both 20% total calories from fat as well as the 1990 US Dietary Guidelines maximum of 30% total calories from fat are provided.

NUTRIENT LABEL CLAIM DEFINITIONS

*Per standard serving size. Some claims have higher nutrient levels for main dish products and meal products, such as frozen entrees and dinners.

Label Claim	Definition
•Good Source, Contains, Provides	10-19% of the Daily Value
•High, Rich In, Excellent Source Of	20% or more of Daily Value
•Fortified, Enriched, Added	Contains at least 10% more of the Daily Value, compared to the reference food

CALORIE-RELATED CLAIMS

•Calorie-free	less than 5 calories
•Low calorie	40 calories or less
•Reduced calorie	At least 25% fewer calories
•Light or lite	At least 1/3 fewer calories or 50% less fat

FAT-RELATED CLAIMS

•Fat-free	Less than 0.5 grams fat
•Low-fat	3 grams or less fat
•Reduced fat	At least 25% less fat

Label Claim	Definition
•Saturated fat-free	Less than 0.5 grams fat
•Low saturated fat	1 gram or less saturated fat and no more than 15% calories from fat
•Reduced saturated fat	At least 25% less saturated fat

CHOLESTEROL-RELATED CLAIMS

•Cholesterol-free	Less than 2 grams cholesterol and 2 grams or less saturated fat
•Low cholesterol	20 mg. or less cholesterol and 2 grams or less saturated fat
•Reduced cholesterol	At least 25% less cholesterol and 2 grams or less saturated fat

SODIUM-RELATED CLAIMS

•Sodium-free	Less than 5 mg. sodium
•Very low sodium	35 mg. or less sodium
•Low sodium	140 mg. or less sodium
•Reduced sodium	At least 25% less sodium
•Light (or Lite) sodium	50% less sodium than normally used on the food

Label Claim	Definition
•Unsalted or No salt added	No salt added during processing

SUGAR-RELATED CLAIMS*
*Sugars include table sugar (sucrose), milk sugar (lactose), honey, corn sweeteners, high fructose corn syrup, molasses, fruit juice concentrate, maple syrup, brown rice syrup, barley malt.

•No added sugars	None of the above sugars is added during processing. It contains no ingredients that contain added sugar. The product it resembles and substitutes for normally contains added sugars.
•Sugar-free	Less than 1/2 gram sugars
•Reduced sugar	At least 25% less sugar

LEAN/EXTRA LEAN MEAT AND POULTRY CLAIMS
Lean	Less than 10% total fat, less than 4 grams saturated fat, less than 95 mg. cholesterol per reference amount and 100 grams
Extra Lean	Less than 5 grams total fat, less than 2 grams saturated fat, less than 95 mg. cholesterol per reference amount and 100 grams

ORGANICALLY PRODUCED CLAIMS

All products: The total percentage of organic ingredients must be declared on the information panel above the ingredient listing. (Air, water, and salt are not included in the calculation.) The name and address of the certifying agency must be provided on the label next to the information identifying the manufacturer or distributor of the food.

•95%-100% organic	May be labeled as organic on front panel. Ingredients listing will also verify the high percentage of organic ingredients contained within the product.
•50-95% organic	If labeled as organic on front display panel, specific ingredients that are organic must be listed. Ingredients panel must also specify which ingredients are organic.
•less than 50% organic	May make no mention on the front panel of the ingredients being organic. Indication of what ingredients are organic may only be listed on ingredients panel.

HEALTH CLAIMS

Claims are allowed to be used on food labels linking a nutrient or food to the risk of a disease or health-related condition:

•calcium and a lower risk of osteoporosis
•fat and a greater risk of cancer
•saturated fat and cholesterol and a greater risk of coronary heart disease
•fiber-containing grain products, fruits, and vegetables and a reduced risk of cancer
•fruits, vegetables, and grain products that contain fiber and a reduced risk of coronary heart disease
•sodium and a greater risk of high blood pressure
•fruits and vegetables and a reduced risk of cancer

WORDS TO KNOW ABOUT INGREDIENTS AND FOOD PROCESSING

acidulant: acids used in processed foods to contribute or enhance flavor, control microbial growth, change or maintain acidity during processing, help coagulate milk proteins in cheeses/spreads, and control gelling in desserts and jams.

alkali: alkalis used in processed foods to reduce acidity or control alkalinity to contribute or enhance flavor, texture, improve cooking properties, and to preserve.

anticaking agent: makes powdery or crystalline ingredients free-flowing, free from caking, lumping, and clumping.

antifoaming agent: prevents excess foaming during processing or when heated at certain temperatures.

antimycotic agent: prevents the growth of molds.

antioxidant: delays or prevents rancidity and enzymatic browning in foods. In the human body, an antioxidant prevents cells from damage by the chemical reaction known as oxidation. Chemically unstable,

15

naturally occurring oxygen molecules that damage inner and outer cell walls are called free radicals.

artificial sweetener: artificially-derived high-intensity sweeteners ranging from 30-600 times the sweetness of table sugar. Some are calorie-free. Seizures, headaches, mood swings, blurred vision, weight gain, and other problems have been linked as side effects.

binder: a substance that maintains the texture and consistency of foods by preventing mixtures from separating or settling.

biotechnology: the genetic modification of bacteria, plants, insects, fish, or animals in which certain genes for traits viewed as desirable, possibly from other species, are spliced within the gene material to modify species significantly more quickly than natural selection or selective breeding. Several consumer groups and scientists question its safety.

buffer: controls the acidity/alkalinity level within a product.

carcinogen: a substance that can produce cancer in experimental animals or is known to do so in humans.

color retention agent: preserves color and brightness.

colorant: synthetically manufactured or naturally derived sources of color. Synthetic water-soluble colors certified by the FDA are designated as FD & C colors. Certified synthetic water-insoluble colors are referred to as FD & C aluminum lakes. Many artificial colors have been suspected of being toxic or carcinogenic.

dough conditioner: used to aid production or modify the appearance and texture of baked goods.

emulsifier: helps keep liquids and oily substances within a product in suspension to improve consistency, texture, and stability.

enrich: replaces vitamins and minerals lost in processing.

fat substitute: low-calorie fat replacements that simulate the body and creamy texture of fat. While gums, malto-dextrin, and starches have been used safely for years, some of the newer versions are suspect.

firming agent: helps preserve the firmness and texture of cut fruits and vegetables.

flavor enhancer: intensifies, modifies, and accentuates flavors.

flavoring agent: restores flavors lost in processing, intensifies natural flavors. May be naturally derived or artificial.

fortify: adds nutrients to a food to make it richer in nutrients than would be found in the original unprocessed food.

fungicides: chemicals used to kill or suppress the growth of all or individual fungi. Often included under the term "pesticides."

GRAS: abbreviation of "Generally Recognized As Safe," a category of both synthetic and naturally-derived substances that were made exempt from the 1958 legal requirement for formal testing and government approval based on longtime common usage in foods prior to that time. Since 1971, many of the suspect GRAS additives have been undergoing testing for safety. Therefore, placement on the GRAS list is no guarantee that the substance is without question.

herbicides: chemicals used to kill or suppress the growth of certain or all plants. Often included under the term "pesticides."

humectant: helps foods retain moisture.

incidental additives: residues from packaging chemicals, pesticides, and fumigants applied during growing, processing, packaging, or storing of food, including residues from drugs administered to farm animals.

insecticides: chemicals used to kill many or certain insects. Often included under the term "pesticides."

intentional additives: additives intentionally added during food processing to aid production, preserve, season, enhance flavors, add color, texture, stabilize, or modify the appearance of food.

IPM: abbreviation for Integrated Pest Management, a food production method that minimizes dependence upon chemicals through physical, cultural, biological, genetic, and preventative means. Pesticides and herbicides remain an option.

irradiation: a process in which food is exposed to gamma radiation from radioactive materials such as cobalt-60, cesium-137, or through linear accelerator electron beams to kill bacteria, insects, or parasites that may be present in food. Significant nutrient losses occur in the process, as well as the potential for the formation of new unknown compounds, commonly referred to as unique radiolytic products.

leavening agent: biological or chemical-based substance that helps produce carbon dioxide which, in turn, increases the volume and lightens the texture in baked goods.

lubricant: prevents food from sticking to machinery during production.

maturing/bleaching agent: accelerates the aging process in flour, improves baking qualities, and whitens the flour's color.

nutrient: supplies vitamins or minerals to enrich or fortify a food.

organically grown: produced according to the requirements of the Federal organic certification program using management-intensive methods designed to promote and enhance soil fertility, biological cycles, and biodiversity. No prohibited fertilizers, chemical pesticides, herbicides, or fungicides may have been applied for at least 3 years prior to marketing as organic. Organic foods are processed, packaged, transported, and stored to retain maximum nutritional value, without the use of artificial preservatives or colorings, irradiation, or toxic synthetic pesticides.

pesticides: chemicals used to control insects, weeds, fungi, rodents, and other unwanted pests during crop production and storage.

pH control agents: substances that are added to change or maintain acidity or alkalinity.

preservative: a substance used to prevent spoilage from bacteria, molds, fungi, and yeast to extend shelf life and protect colors and flavors.

rodenticide: chemical used to control rodents or related animals, such as gophers. Often included under the term "pesticides."

sequestrant: chemicals added to food to bind minerals, such as calcium, iron, and copper, that can oxidize and cause staleness, rancidity, off-flavors and discoloration.

stabilizer: a substance that maintains the texture and consistency of foods by preventing mixtures from separating or settling.

stimulant: a substance that affects the central nervous system, increasing the heart beat and the basal metabolic rate.

sweetener: an ingredient added to foods to enhance the flavor. See also "artificial sweetener."

synergistic effect: the tendency of chemicals acting in combination with one another to produce effects greater than the sum of the effects of individual chemicals.

texturizer: improves the texture of a processed food.

thickener: provides body and thicker consistency in a processed food.

whipping agent: helps increase and sustain the volume in foods.

While, technically, any ingredient listed on a label is approved for food use by the government, it is no guarantee that the substance is without risk. Currently sophisticated analysis techniques are better able to ascertain safety; therefore, some ingredients approved in the past are now suspect of being harmful to health. In some foods, the overuse of additives has created a food that looks and perhaps tastes like the original but dramatically reduces its nutritional content.

Always opt for products with the least complex ingredient labels which list food items rather than synthesized additives. A general rule of thumb is to avoid any product with artificial flavors, artificial colors, artificial preservatives, and artificial sweeteners. Products too high in fat and sweeteners should also be avoided. To help you avoid these and other questionable ingredients, you'll find a specific list of additives to avoid within each food group detailed in this book.

BREAD, CEREAL, RICE, & PASTA GROUP

WORDS TO KNOW ABOUT GRAINS

aflatoxin: a carcinogenic toxin produced by a fungus, Aspergillus flavus, that can grow on grains, nuts, and peanuts. It grows best on plants that are weakened by insects or stressed from the lack of moisture during a drought.

bleaching and maturing agents: chemicals used to accelerate the aging process for flour and also to improve baking qualities.

desem: a type of sourdough culture that is produced from the interaction of organisms and enzymes that naturally occur in wheat flour instead of relying on airborne yeasts and bacteria.

dough conditioners: additives used to aid production or modify the appearance and texture of the final baked product.

enrichment: the addition of nutrients back to a food to meet a standard or to restore nutrients lost in processing. By law, any bread or cereal labeled as "enriched" must include added thiamin, riboflavin, niacin, iron, and folic acid.

gluten: a protein complex that provides the elastic properties in bread doughs and the appearance and structure of baked goods. Some individuals are sensitive to gluten, causing them digestive difficulties.

leavened breads: breads leavened with baking yeast and/or sourdough.

lime treatment of corn: an alkalizing treatment with calcium chloride (slaked lime) to help remove the corn's tough outer hull for easier eating and processing. It also improves the amino acid balance, liberates the bound niacin, and provides calcium.

mochi: a traditional Japanese food made from steamed and mashed sweet rice dried in shallow pans and cut into squares. When baked in a 450° F. oven, broiled, or pan-fried for 10 minutes, mochi puffs up into delicious, chewy "biscuits."

organically grown: certified to be produced according to the requirements of the Federal organic certification program using management-intensive methods designed to promote and enhance soil fertility, biological cycles, and biodiversity. No prohibited fertilizers, chemical pesticides, herbicides, or fungicides may have been applied for at least 3 years prior to marketing as organic. Organic foods are processed, packaged, transported, and stored to retain maximum nutritional value, without the use of artificial preservatives or colorings, irradiation, or toxic synthetic chemicals.

quick breads: breads leavened with baking soda, baking powder, and/or eggs. Free of baking yeast and sourdough.

refined grains: grains that have been processed of much of their fiber and, usually, their germ, resulting in significantly less nutrients than are found in whole grains.

seitan: a concentrated source of protein made by cooking the gluten extracted from wheat flour within a broth made from soy sauce and kombu (a sea vegetable). Its chewy texture and full-bodied flavor are similar to roast beef and it is just as versatile.

WHOLE GRAINS BUYING GUIDE

1 lb. GRAIN	GLUTEN?	UNCOOKED	COOKED YIELDS
amaranth	no	2 1/2 cups	6 1/4 cups
barley	yes	pearled: 2 1/3 cups whole: 2 1/3 cups flakes: 4 cups	8 cups 8 cups 14 cups
buckwheat	no	2 3/4 cups	7 cups

sourdough: natural leavening resulting from the interaction of bacteria and wild yeasts found naturally in the air with a thick mixture of flour and water. Sometimes labeled yeast-free.

stone-ground: a method of grinding flour in which the flour is ground between two flat millstones that rub against each other. The stones slowly crush the grain, distributing its bran and nutrient-rich germ throughout the flour.

whole grains: grains that retain their bran and germ along with their endosperm. Whole grains contain significantly more nutrients and fiber than refined grains.

STORAGE/COOKING	WHAT TO DO WITH IT
6 months at room temp. Cooks in 20-25 minutes.	Strong, nutty spicy flavor and gelatinous texture; best cooked with other grains.
12 months at room temp. 6 months storage for flakes. Pearled: cooks in 60 minutes. Whole:cooks in 90 minutes. Flakes: cooks in 25 minutes.	Use in salads, pilafs, or to thicken soups/stews.
6 months at room temp. Cooks in 15-20 minutes.	Use in pilafs and cereals.

WHOLE GRAINS BUYING GUIDE

1 lb. GRAIN	GLUTEN?	UNCOOKED	COOKED YIELDS
bulgur wheat	yes	2 3/4 cups	7 cups
cornmeal	no	3 1/2 cups	10 1/2 cups
couscous	yes	2 7/8 cups	8 2/3 cups
cracked wheat	yes	3 cups	7 cups
kamut	yes	whole: 2 1/2 cups	7 1/2 cups
		flakes: 3 2/3 cups	9 cups
millet	no	2 1/3 cups	8 cups
oats	yes	rolled: 4 1/4 cups	10 2/3 cups
		steel-cut: 2 3/4 cups	8 1/4 cups
		whole: 2 3/4 cups	8 1/4 cups
quinoa	no	2 7/8 cups	10 cups

STORAGE/COOKING

6 months at room temp.
Cooks in 15-20 minutes
or soak in boiling water
for one hour.

3 months in refrigerator
Cooks in 25-30 minutes.

6 months at room temp.
Cooks in 5-10 minutes.

3 months in refrigerator.
Cooks in 20 minutes.

6 months at room temp.
Whole: cooks in 90 minutes
or 35 minutes if pre-soaked.
Flakes: cook in 18 minutes.

6 months at room temp.
Cooks in 30 minutes.

12 months at room temp.
Rolled oats: cooks in 10-15
minutes. Steel-cut cooks in
30 minutes. Whole cooks in
90 minutes.

3 months at room temp.
Cooks in 15 minutes.

WHAT TO DO WITH IT

Use in tabouli salad, cereals,
and as a ground beef substitute in chili.

Use as cereal or to make
polenta.

Use in salads, pilafs, desserts,
or as a cereal.

Use as cereal, in salads,
casseroles, and pilafs.

Use in salads, cereals,
or to extend soups, stews,
and chilis.

Use in pilafs, stuffings,
salads, casseroles, and
croquettes.

Use in cereals, pilafs,
stews, and casseroles.

Use in pilafs and cereals.

WHOLE GRAINS BUYING GUIDE

1 lb. GRAIN	GLUTEN?	UNCOOKED	COOKED YIELDS
rice	no	white: 2 1/2 cups brown: 2 3/4 cups	7 cups 8 cups
rye	yes	whole: 2 1/3 cups flakes: 4 cups	8 cups 12 cups
spelt	yes	whole: 2 1/2 cups flakes: 4 1/3 cups	7 1/2 cups 10 3/4 cups
teff	no	2 1/4 cups	6 3/4 cups
triticale	yes	whole: 2 1/3 cups flakes: 4 cups	7 cups 9 cups

STORAGE/COOKING

3 months (brown rice)
12 months (white rice)
Short & med. brown:
cooks in 50 minutes. Short
white cooks in 15 minutes.
Arborio cooks in 25 minutes.
Long brown cooks in 45
minutes. Long white: cooks
in 15 minutes.

6 months room temp.
Whole: cooks in 1-2 hours.
Flakes: cooks in 25-30 minutes.

6 months at room temp.
Flakes: 3 months at room temp.
Whole: cooks in 90 minutes or
in 1 hour if pre-soaked. Flakes:
cooks in 18-20 minutes.

6 months at room temp.
Cooks in 15 minutes.

6 months at room temp.
Whole: cooks in 90 minutes
or 50 minutes if presoaked.
Flakes: cooks in 15-20 minutes.

WHAT TO DO WITH IT

Use in pilafs, cereals,
salads, and casseroles.

Use in pilafs, cereals,
and casseroles.

Use in pilafs, cereals,
and casseroles.

Use in cereals, desserts,
and prepared like polenta.

Use in pilafs, cereals,
and casseroles.

WHOLE GRAINS BUYING GUIDE

1 lb. GRAIN	GLUTEN?	UNCOOKED	COOKED YIELDS
wheat	yes	whole: 2 1/3 cups	7 cups
		flakes: 4 cups	9 cups
		germ: 4 cups	not applicable
wild rice	no	2 cups	8 cups

BREAKFAST CEREAL BUYING GUIDE

Look for
• whole grains ground, rolled, flaked, shredded, or puffed
• at least a moderate amount of dietary fiber, about 3-4 grams.
• a simple sugar content less than 4 grams per serving (equivalent to 1 teaspoon sugar. Avoid any cereal that lists sugar, honey, corn syrup, fructose, molasses, fruit juice sweetener, or malt syrup as the first ingredient.)
• less than 140 mg. sodium per serving

STORAGE/COOKING

6 months at room temp.
wheat germ: 7 days in fridge.
Whole: cooks in 90 minutes or
50 minutes if pre-soaked.
Flakes: cooks in 30 minutes.

12 months at room temp.
Cooks in 60 minutes or mix
equally with brown rice and
cook 45 minutes.

WHAT TO DO WITH IT

Use in pilafs, cereals,
salads, casseroles, and.
to extend soups, stews,
and chilis.

Use in pilafs, salads,
and casseroles.

STORAGE GUIDELINES FOR CEREALS

TYPE	UNOPENED	OPENED
ready-to-eat*	6-12 months	3 months
hot cereals, uncooked	12 months	6 months, best in fridge
hot cereal, cooked	N/A	3-4 days in fridge
granola	6 months	6 months, best in fridge

*check dating on box

CEREAL ADDITIVES TO AVOID

artificial color
artificial flavor
artificial sweeteners
BHA (antioxidant, preservative)
BHT (in packaging—antioxidant, preservative)
partially hydrogenated oil (treated to prolong shelf
   life and to provide texture and body)
TBHQ (antioxidant, preservative)

FLOUR BUYING GUIDE

1 LB. FLOUR	GLUTEN?	YIELD	FLAVOR
amaranth	no	3 1/2 cups	strong, spicy
arrowroot	no	3 1/2 cups	neutral
barley	yes	3 1/3 cups	sweet, malty
buckwheat	no	3 3/4 cups	hearty
chickpea	no	3 1/2 cups	sweet, rich
cornmeal	no	3 1/4 cups	sweet, nutty
gluten	yes	3 1/4 cups	tangy

GRANOLA BARS/BREAKFAST BARS
ADDITIVES TO AVOID

artificial color

artificial flavor

BHT (antioxidant, preservative)

partially hydrogenated oil (treated to prolong shelf
   life and to provide texture and body)

potassium sorbate (preservative, antimycotic agent)

sulfur dioxide (preservative, antioxidant, color
   retention agent)

TBHQ (antioxidant, preservative)

BAKED TEXTURE	STORAGE
smooth, crisp crust moist, fine crumb	3 months cool room 6 months in fridge
lightens wheat-free baked goods	3 months cool room 6 months in fridge
firm, chewy crust cakelike crumb	3 months cool room 6 months in fridge
moist, fine crumb	3 months cool room 6 months in fridge
dry, delicate crumb	3 months cool room 6 months in fridge
grainy, slightly dry	always refrigerate up to 6 months
fine crumb crisp, thin crust	3 months cool room 6 months in fridge

FLOUR BUYING GUIDE

1 LB. FLOUR	GLUTEN?	YIELD	FLAVOR
kamut	yes	3 1/4 cups	rich, buttery
millet	no	3 cups	mildly sweet, buttery
oat	yes	4 1/2 cups	sweet, nutty
potato	no	3 cups	sweetly pungent
quinoa	no	3 2/3 cups	nutty
rice	no	3 cups	nutty
rye	yes	4 cups	tangy
soy	no	4 cups	slightly bitter
spelt	yes	3 1/4 cups	sweet, nutty
teff	no	3 cups	sweet, malty
triticale	yes	3 1/2 cups	nutty, tangy
wheat, unbleached white	yes	3 1/2 cups	nutty, bland
whole wheat	yes	3 1/2 cups	sweet, nutty
whole wheat pastry	no	4 cups	sweet, nutty

BAKED TEXTURE	STORAGE
dense, heavy crumb	3 months cool room 6 months in fridge
dry, delicate crumb smooth, thin crust	always refrigerate up to 3 months
moist, cakelike crumb, firm crust	3 months cool room 6 months in fridge
soft, dry crust fine, springy crumb	3 months cool room 6 months in fridge
delicate, cakelike crumb	always refrigerate up to 3 months
dry, fine crumb	3 months cool room 6 months in fridge
moist, crumb smooth, hard crust	3 month cool room 6 months in fridge
moist, fine crumb smooth, hard crust	3 months cool room 6 months in fridge
moderate crumb supple crust	3 months cool room 6 months in fridge
delicate crumb	3 months cool room 6 months in fridge
dense crumb semi-firm crust	3 months cool room 6 months in fridge
fine crumb	6 months cool room
coarse, large crumb	3 months cool room 6 months in fridge
fine crumb	3 months cool room 6 months in fridge

FLOUR ADDITIVES TO AVOID

bleached flour
bromated flour
calcium peroxide

BAKING MIX ADDITIVES TO AVOID

artificial color
artificial flavor
artificial sweeteners
BHT (antioxidant, preservative)
bleached flour (artificially aged)
partially hydrogenated oil (treated to prolong shelf
    life and to provide texture and body)
potassium sorbate (preservative, antimycotic agent)
sodium benzoate (antimycotic agent)
sulfur dioxide (preservative, antioxidant, color
    retention agent)
TBHQ (antioxidant, preservative)

MUFFIN/SNACK CAKES ADDITIVES TO AVOID

artificial color
artificial flavor
bleached flour (artificially aged)
calcium peroxide (dough conditioner, bleaching agent)
calcium propionate (antimycotic agent)
partially hydrogenated oil (treated to prolong shelf
    life and to provide texture and body)
potassium sorbate (preservative, antimycotic agent)
sodium propionate (antimycotic agent)
stearoyl-2-lactylate (dough conditioner)

BREADS

Look for:
- whole grain flour
- simple ingredients list, with little more than flour, water, salt, and a leavening agent
- preferably 2-3 grams of fiber per slice
- minimal sweeteners, preferably none

Yields/equivalents

1 lb. loaf	12-16 slices
1 slice	approx. 1/2 cup soft crumbs
1 slice	approx. 1/3 cup dry crumbs
1 cup soft crumbs	2/3 cup dry crumbs
4 ounces	2 cups cubed

HOW TO STORE BREAD

(average length of time based on breads free of preservatives)

TYPE	BEST STORAGE	HOW LONG	FREEZER STORAGE
hard-crusted: yeasted breads sourdough breads	room temperature loosely wrapped in paper, towel, perforated cellophane bag in bread box or countertop.	2-3 days	3 months
soft crusted yeasted breads	room temperature tightly closed plastic bag. Up to 7 days in fridge.	2-4 days	4 months

HOW TO STORE BREAD

(average length of time based on breads free of preservatives)

TYPE	BEST STORAGE	HOW LONG	FREEZER STORAGE
quick breads	room temperature tightly closed plastic bag. Up to 7 days in fridge.	2 days	3 months
pita bread	room temperature tightly closed plastic bag. Up to 7 days in fridge.	2 days	4 months
tortillas	room temperature tightly closed plastic bag. Up to 7 days in fridge.	2 days	4 months
crackers	room temperature tightly wrapped.	6 months unopened 1 month open	N/A

WHEAT-FREE BREADS

(ready-made alternatives for individuals sensitive/
   allergic to wheat)

corn tortillas   rice cakes   spelt bagels**
kamut bread**   rice crackers   spelt bread**
millet bread   rye bread*
rice bread   rye crackers*

*some individuals allergic to wheat are also allergic to rye and other
   grains that contain gluten.
**some individuals allergic to wheat may tolerate kamut and spelt,
   two varieties of ancient strains of wheat

BREAD, TORTILLAS, & CRACKER ADDITIVES TO AVOID

artificial color

artificial flavor

azodicarbonamide (ADA) (dough conditioner)

bleached flour (artificially aged)

calcium disodium EDTA (antioxidant, sequestrant)

calcium peroxide (dough conditioner, bleaching agent)

calcium propionate (antimycotic agent)

carboxymethyl cellulose gum (thickener, binder, stabilizer)

L-cysteine (shortcut method, yielding mediocre bread)

lactic acid in sourdough breads (harmless but mediocre flavor imitator of sourdough)

monosodium glutamate (MSG) (flavor enhancer)

partially hydrogenated oil (treated to prolong shelf life and to provide texture and body)

potassium bromate (dough conditioner, flour maturing agent)

potassium sorbate (preservative, antimycotic agent)

sodium benzoate (preservative, antimycotic agent)

sodium diacetate in sourdough breads (harmless but mediocre flavor imitator of sourdough)

sodium propionate (antimycotic agent)

sodium stearoyl lactylate (shortcut method yielding mediocre bread)

stearoyl-2-lactylate (shortcut method yielding mediocre bread)

BREAD STUFFING MIX ADDITIVES TO AVOID

azodicarbonamide (dough conditioner)
BHT (antioxidant, preservative)
calcium propionate (antimycotic)
disodium guanylate (flavor enhancer)

PASTA BUYING GUIDE

1 LB. PASTA	UNCOOKED	COOKED YIELDS
egg noodles	7-8 cups*	8 cups
fresh pasta	6 cups	6 cups
jerusalem artichoke pasta	macaroni: 3 3/4 cups	8 cups
	noodles: 6-8 cups*	8 cups
	shells: 4-5 cups	9 cups
	spaghetti: 3" diameter	8-9 cups
	spirals: 5-6 cups	6-7 cups
kamut pasta	noodles: 6-8 cups*	8 cups
	spirals: 7 cups	8 cups
lupini pasta	macaroni: 4 cups	9 cups
	noodles: 6-8 cups*	8 cups
	spaghetti: 3" diameter	7-8 cups

*Note: Uncooked noodle measure is based on uncrushed noodles. Some brands are less flat and, therefore, may have a higher cup volume than indicated on this chart.

disodium inosinate (flavor enhancer)
monosodium glutamate (flavor enhancer)
partially hydrogenated oil (treated to prolong
   shelf life and to provide texture and body)
sodium sulfite (preservative, antioxidant, color
   retention agent)

STORAGE/COOKING	WHAT TO DO WITH IT
Store up to 6 months at room temperature. Cooks in 5-7 minutes.	Toss with mildly flavored, light sauces. Good in casseroles.
1-2 days in fridge. Cooks in 1-3 minutes.	Toss with oil, pesto, or a light sauce.
Store up to 18 months at room temperature. Cooks in 4-10 minutes.	Toss with oil, pesto, light or hearty sauces.
Store up to 6 months at room temperature. Cooks in 4-10 minutes.	Toss with oil, pesto, light or hearty sauces, beans, tofu, tempeh, fish, poultry.
Store up to 18 months at room temperature. Cooks in 8-10 minutes.	Toss with pesto, light or hearty sauces, beans, tofu, tempeh, fish, poultry. Cooked pasta keeps loose and separate without the need for oil.

PASTA BUYING GUIDE

1 LB. PASTA	UNCOOKED	COOKED YIELDS
orzo	2 2/3 cups	5-6 cups
semolina pasta	macaroni: 3 3/4 cups	8 cups
	noodles: 6-8 cups*	8 cups
	penne: 5 1/2 cups	8 1/2 cups
	shells: 4-5 cups	9 cups
	spaghetti: 3" diameter	8-9 cups
	spirals: 5-6 cups	6 cups
sesame-rice pasta (also contains wheat)	spirals: 5-6 cups	6 cups
spelt pasta	macaroni: 4 cups	9 cups
	spirals: 8 cups (spaghetti tends to fall apart)	9 cups
whole wheat pasta	macaroni: 3 3/4 cups	9 cups
	noodles: 6-8 cups*	8 cups
	shells: 4-5 cups	9 cups
	spaghetti: 3" diameter	8-9 cups
	spirals: 6 cups	8 cups

ORIENTAL NOODLES

bifun noodles (white rice flour and potato starch)	16 cups (these are very light weight noodles)	16 cups

STORAGE/COOKING	WHAT TO DO WITH IT
Store up to 18 months at room temperature. Cooks in 4-6 minutes.	Serve as accompaniment to meal like rice or combine with veggies and dressing for a salad.
Store up to 18 months at room temperature. Cooks in 4-10 minutes.	Its bland flavor makes it a good choice as a background when the sauce or entree is the focal point of the meal.
Store up to 12 months. at room temperature. Cooks in 8-10 minutes.	Toss with oil or light sauce, beans, tofu, tempeh, fish.
Store up to 12 months at room temperature. Cooks in 8-10 minutes.	Toss with oil, light or hearty sauces, beans, tofu, tempeh, fish, poultry.
Store up to 1 year at room temperature. Cooks in 4-10 minutes	Toss with oil, pesto, light and hearty sauces, beans, tofu, tempeh, fish, poultry.
Store up to 18 months at room temperature. Cooks in 5-6 minutes or soak in hot water for 10-20 minutes.	Use in salads, clear soups, sukiyaki, and fried noodle dishes.

PASTA BUYING GUIDE

1 LB. PASTA	UNCOOKED	COOKED YIELDS
kuzu kiri (kuzu and potato starch)	16" diameter (these are very light weight noodles)	8 cups
ramen	sold in individual blocks with seasoning packet. Avoid varieties made with monosodium glutamate and artificial flavoring.	serves 1-2
rice sticks	16" diameter	8 cups
saifun noodles (mung bean starch)	16 cups (these are very light weight noodles)	16 cups
soba (buckwheat and usually wheat)	3" diameter	6 1/3 cups
somen	3" diameter	7-8 cups
udon	3" diameter	8 cups

STORAGE/COOKING	WHAT TO DO WITH IT
Store up to 18 months at room temperature. Cooks in 20 minutes.	Use in sukiyaki, salads, or served in a light broth.
Store up to 6 months at room temperature. Cooks in 6 minutes.	Serve as is or add extra veggies and tofu, cooked tempeh, or cooked fish or poultry.
Store up to 18 months at room temperature. Cooks in 1-5 minutes or soak in water 15 minutes and then stir-fry.	Use in soups, cold noodle dishes, stir-fries, Pad Thai.
Store up to 18 months at room temperature. Cooks in 5-6 minutes or soak in hot water for 10-20 minutes.	Use in salads, clear soups, sukiyaki, and fried noodle dishes.
Store up to 12 months at room temperature. Cooks in 5-8 minutes.	Use in salads or toss with oil, light sauce, beans, tofu, tempeh, fish. Mugwort soba has spinach-like flavor. Jinenjo has nutty flavor.
Store up to 18 months at room temperature. Cooks in 4-6 minutes.	Serve cold in salads or toss with oil or light sauce and veggies.
Store up to 18 months at room temperature. Cooks in 5-8 minutes.	Toss with oil, light sauce or hearty sauce, beans, tofu, tempeh, fish, poultry.

PASTA BUYING GUIDE

1 LB. PASTA	UNCOOKED	COOKED YIELDS
WHEAT-FREE PASTAS		
brown rice pasta	spirals: 8 cups	8 cups
	spaghetti: 3 1/2" diameter	8-9 cups
corn pasta	macaroni: 4 cups	6 cups
	shells: 4-5 cups	9 cups
	spaghetti: 3 1/2" diameter	8-9 cups

PASTA ADDITIVES TO AVOID
(Generally, additives in pasta found only in ramen)
monosodium glutamate (MSG) (flavor enhancer)
disodium guanylate (flavor enhancer)
disodium inosinate (flavor enhancer)
partially hydrogenated oil (treated to prolong
    shelf life and to provide texture and body)

STORAGE/COOKING	WHAT TO DO WITH IT
Store up to 12 months at room temperature. Cooks in 4-5 minutes.	Toss with oil, light sauce, beans, tofu, tempeh, fish, poultry.
Store up to 12 months at room temperature. Cooks in 4-5 minutes.	Toss with oil, hearty sauce, beans, tofu, tempeh.

WORDS TO KNOW ABOUT VEGETABLES

biotechnology: the genetic modification of bacteria, plants, insects, fish, or animals in which certain genes for traits viewed as desirable, possibly from other species, are spliced within the gene material to modify species significantly more quickly than natural selection or selective breeding. Several consumer groups and scientists question its safety in the long run.

conventionally grown: food which may be grown with the aid of pesticides, herbicides, and fungicides.

cruciferous vegetables: a family of vegetables that contain compounds which help stimulate the production of protective enzymes that detoxify potential carcinogens. They are named as such because the flowers that bloom from the plants have four petals that form the shape of a cross. Includes: arugula, bok choy, broccoli, brussels sprouts, cabbage, cauliflower, collard greens, kale, mustard greens, radishes, turnips.

IPM: Integrated Pest Management: production methods that minimize dependence on pesticides, herbicides, and fertilizers by employing physical, cultural, biological, genetic, and preventatve measures. While IPM is a step in the right direction, it is no guarantee that the product is grown without agricultural chemicals.

organically grown: certified to be produced according to the requirements of the National Organic Standards using management-intensive methods designed to promote and enhance soil fertility, biological cycles, and biodiversity. No prohibited fertilizers, chemical pesticides, herbicides, or fungicides may have been applied for at least 3 years prior to marketing as organic. Organic foods are processed, packaged, transported, and stored to retain maximum nutritional value, without the use of artificial preservatives or colorings, irradiation, or toxic synthetic chemicals.

sea vegetables: plants cultivated from sea waters that are used as a source of nourishment for humans.

sprouts: the very young shoots from the germinated seeds of vegetables, beans, or grains for use fresh in salads or lightly cooked (if sprouted beans or grains).

transitional organic: a claim used to signify food produced in which all conditions for organic certification have been met, except for the required three-year length of time for the acreage/product in question to have been free of prohibited inputs or applications.

waxed vegetables: vegetables coated with a variety of waxes to help prevent moisture loss and reduce wilting and shriveling. Many question whether waxes have been thoroughly researched to be safe for consumption. Fungicides may also be mixed in with the wax.

FRESH VEGETABLES BUYING GUIDE

1 lb. veggie	raw yield
artichoke, Jerusalem	3 cups cubed
asparagus	16-20 spears
beets	2 cups
broccoli, flowers/stems	5-6 cups
brussel's sprouts	4 cups
cabbage	6 cups (shredded)
carrots	3 cups (sliced, diced)
cauliflower	1 1/2 cups
celery	1 bunch
corn (4 ears)	2 cups
eggplant, diced	4 cups
green beans	3 cups
green onion (1 bunch)	3/4 cup sliced
greens (kale, collards)	12 cups
lettuce, leaf	8 cups
mushrooms	4 cups sliced
okra	3 1/2 cups
onion	3 large
parsnips	4 medium
peas, in pods	1 cup shelled
pepper, green/red	3 medium
plantain	2 cups pieces
potatoes	3 medium
pumpkin	3 cups cubed
radishes	5 cups sliced
rutabaga	2 1/2 cups cubed
spinach	8 cups
sprouts, alfalfa/mung	6 cups
squash, winter	3 cups cubed
squash, summer	3 cups
sweet potatoes	3 medium
tomatoes	3-4 small
turnips	3 medium

*Leave corn husks on and refrigerate unwrapped.
**Loosely wrap in a paper bag.

cooked yield	uncooked (raw) storage
3 cups	fridge: 1-2 weeks
2 cups	fridge.: 2-3 days
2 cups	fridge: up to 2 weeks
5-6 cups	fridge: 3-4 days
2 1/2 cups	fridge: 3-4 days
2-3 cups	fridge: up to 2 weeks
2 1/4 cups	fridge: up to 2 weeks
1 1/2 cups	fridge: 3-6 days
2 1/4 cups	fridge: 7-10 days
2 cups	fridge: 1-2 days*
1 3/4 cups	fridge: 3-5 days
2 1/2 cups	fridge: 1-2 days
1/4 cup	fridge: 3-5 days
3 cups	fridge: 2-4 days
N/A	fridge: 3-4 days
2 1/2 cups	fridge: 4-5 days**
2 1/4 cups	fridge: 3-4 days
2 cups	cool area: 1-4 weeks
2 1/2 cups	fridge: up to 2 weeks
1 cup	fridge: 3-4 days
2 1/2-3 cups	fridge: 3-5 days
1 1/2 cups	fridge: 3-5 days***
2 1/4 cups	cool area: 1-4 weeks
1 cup mashed	cool area: 1-4 weeks
N/A	fridge: 1-2 weeks
2 cups	fridge: 1-2 weeks
2 cups	fridge: 2-3 days
3 cups (mung only)	fridge: 3-5 days
1 cup mashed	cool area: 1-4 weeks
1 1/2 cups	fridge: 3-5 days
2 cups	cool area: 2 weeks
1 1/2 cups	fridge: 2-4 days***
2 cups	fridge: 5-7 days

*** Ripen at room temperature before refrigerating.

Storage Hints

Unless stated otherwise above, store veggies in a plastic bag in the refrigerator or in the refrigerator crisper (if crisper is kept 2/3 full). Potatoes, sweet potatoes, onions, and winter squashes store best at cool temperatures (50-60° F.) At room temperature, storage time is cut in half.

VEGETABLE JUICE BUYING GUIDE

Choosing the Best Buy for Nutrition
(listed in descending order of nutrient value)

1. freshly extracted juice
2. fresh frozen juice
3. frozen concentrate
4. canned, bottled, or aseptic-packed juice
5. chilled extracted juice

STORAGE GUIDELINES

TYPE	UNOPENED	AFTER OPENING
freshly extracted	N/A	1-2 days fridge
bottled/canned	1 year shelf	7-10 days fridge
juice boxes	6-9 months shelf	7-10 days fridge
frozen juices	8-12 months freezer	7-10 days fridge

5 GOOD REASONS TO CHOOSE ORGANICALLY PRODUCED FOODS

1. Helps protect our water resources
Since harmful synthetic fertilizers and pesticides are not allowed in organic production, the amount of nitrates and toxins which leach into the groundwater is greatly reduced.

2. Reduces health risks
Many pesticides, herbicides, and fertilizers are potential carcinogens, endangering the health of farm workers as well as consumers. Organic production methods rely instead on proper tillage, crop rotation, and manuring.

3. Builds soil health
Building nutrient-rich soil is the foundation of organic agriculture, resulting in soil which resists topsoil erosion—a significant problem we're facing due to current chemical-intensive, mono-crop farming.

4. Helps maintain balance in nature
Organic agriculture respects diversity within the environment, including the protection of plant and wildlife habitat.

5. Organically produced food tastes great
Strong, healthy plants provide optimum flavor as do organically fed livestock allowed to live in conditions that support expression of natural behaviors.

FRESH/FROZEN/CANNED/DRIED VEGETABLE ADDITIVES TO AVOID

added sweeteners

artificial color

artificial flavor

BHT (antioxidant, preservative)

calcium disodium EDTA (antioxidant, sequestrant)

disodium guanylate (flavor enhancer)

disodium inosinate (flavor enhancer)

irradiation (preservation process labeled by phrase "treated by irradiation" as well as the flower-like international irradiation logo)

pesticides/herbicides (buy organically grown fresh and processed veggies whenever possible)

sodium bisulfite (preservative, antioxidant, color retention agent)

wax coatings (cucumbers, eggplants, parsnips, peppers, pumpkins, rutabagas, squash, sweet potatoes, turnips)

PEAK SEASONS FOR VEGETABLES

Domestically grown produce purchased during its optimum growing season is always the best buy. Locally grown is even better since transportation time to the store is minimal, increasing the likelihood that it is more fresh, retaining more nutrients. Out-of-season vegetables are generally more costly and less flavorful. Imported produce often contains more pesticides than domestically grown produce, possibly pesticides that are banned for use in the United States. Imported produce may also be fumigated before it is allowed to enter the country.

The best produce departments will have both the growing method and country of origin clearly displayed for each type of vegetable. Only then can you make reasonable, informed choices.

JANUARY/FEBRUARY
broccoli
cabbage
carrots
celery
collard greens
fennel
kale
leeks
mushrooms
mustard greens
rutabaga
spinach
winter squash

MARCH, APRIL, MAY
artichokes
asparagus
broccoli
cabbage
carrots
collard greens
dandelion greens
leeks
mustard greens
peas
new potatoes
sorrel
spinach
watercress

JUNE, JULY, AUGUST
arugula
asparagus (June)
beets
cabbage
carrots
chard
corn
cucumbers
eggplant
garlic
green beans
fava beans
kohlrabi
lima beans
okra
pattypan squashes
peppers
radishes
sorrel
spaghetti squash
yellow summer squash
zucchini

SEPTEMBER, OCTOBER, NOVEMBER, DECEMBER

arugula
beets
Belgian endive
broccoli
brussels sprouts
cabbage
carrots
cauliflower
celery root
chard
fennel
garlic
kale
leeks
mushrooms
mustard greens
parsley
peppers
snow peas
potatoes
pumpkin
rutabaga
sweet potatoes
yams
winter squash

HOW TO MINIMIZE EXPOSURE TO PESTICIDE RESIDUES

1. Buy certified organically grown whenever possible.

2. Wash all produce in water before consuming or preparing. A diluted solution of dishwashing soap and water may remove some surface pesticide residues. Systemic pesticides that have been incorporated within the vegetable will not be removed.

3. Peel waxed produce. Vegetable wax or food-grade shellacs may be applied to produce to seal in moisture and extend shelf life. It also seals in agricultural chemicals that may have been applied to the produce. Washing will not remove waxes. (By law, grocery stores are required to label produce that has been waxed.) Unfortunately peeling also reduces nutrient value as well as fiber.

SPROUTS

Sprouts are nutritionally comparable to lettuce. Some
stores grow their own in trays ready for you to harvest
while other stores are supplied by local vendors on a
frequent basis. In either case, before you buy sprouts,
make sure they look very fresh, with no evident wilting or root rot. Sprouts labeled as certified organic must
be grown from organic seeds. Sprouts are also very easy
to grow yourself. See *Good Food: The Complete Guide to
Eating Well* for detailed instructions.

SEA VEGETABLES AT A GLANCE

TYPE	STORAGE/COOKING	WHAT TO DO WITH IT
agar	Keeps indefinitely in cool, dry, dark place. Cooks in 10 minutes.	Use as gelling agent for vegetarian gelatin-type desserts, aspics, puddings, pie fillings.
alaria	Keeps indefinitely in cool, dry, dark place. Cooks in 20 minutes.	Cook with soups, stews, and with grains.
arame	Keeps indefinitely in cool, dry, dark place. Cooks in 30 minutes.	Add to vegetable sautés and casseroles.
dulse	Keeps indefinitely in cool, dark, dry place Cooks in 5 minutes. Can be eaten raw.	Add to chowder, stews, salads, and sandwiches.

SEA VEGETABLES AT A GLANCE

TYPE	STORAGE/COOKING	WHAT TO DO WITH IT
hijiki	Keeps indefinitely in cool, dark, dry place. Cooks in 30 minutes.	Add to casseroles, soups, stews, noodle dishes, and salads.
kelp	Keeps indefinitely in cool, dark, dry place. Cooks in 20 minutes. Often sold granulated.	Use granulated as salty condiment. Add Atlantic kelp to soups, stews, stews, and beans.
kombu	Keeps indefinitely in cool, dark, dry place. Cooks in 30 minutes.	Use as a flavor enhancer for soup stocks, broths, stews, and beans.
nori	Keeps indefinitely in cool, dark, dry place. Toast nori over heat for a couple seconds. Dark iridescent green pre-toasted nori is ready to eat.	Use to wrap sushi, nori maki, and rice balls. Crumble or cut nori to garnish soups, salads, grain dishes, noodles, veggies, and casseroles.
sea palm	Keeps indefinitely in cool, dark, dry place. Presoak 20-60 minutes before using.	Add to soups, salads, and sautés.
wakame	Keeps indefinitely in cool, dark, dry place. Soak for salads or cook 5-10 minutes.	Use in salads, soups, and vegetable dishes.

WORDS TO KNOW ABOUT FRUIT

100% juice: unmodified juice that contains the minimum soluble solids content by weight (the Brix level), as set by the government, for the particular juice in question.

conventionally grown: food which may be grown with the aid of pesticides, herbicides, and fungicides.

IPM: Integrated Pest Management: production methods that minimize dependence on pesticides, herbicides, and fertilizers by employing physical, cultural, biological, genetic, and preventatve measures. While IPM is a step in the right direction, it is no guarantee that the product is grown without agricultural chemicals.

modified juice: juice that has had its color, taste, aroma, or other organoleptic properties processed to the extent that it no longer resembles the original juice. Also includes juices whose nutrient profile has been diminished of any essential nutrient that is normally present in a measurable amount. Modified juices used within a juice product must be listed on the ingredients panel with a short description of how it was modified.

organically grown: certified to be produced according to the requirements of the National Organic Standards using management-intensive methods designed to promote and enhance soil fertility, biological cycles, and biodiversity. No prohibited fertilizers, chemical pesticides, herbicides, or fungicides may have been applied for at least 3 years prior to marketing as organic. Foods labeled as organic are processed, packaged, transported, and stored to retain maximum nutritional value, without the use of artificial preservatives or colorings, irradiation, or toxic synthetic chemicals.

sulfites/sulfur dioxide: the application of sulfur dioxide, sodium sulfite, sodium and potassium bisulfite, or sodium and potassium metabisulfite to retain moisture and color of the fruit. Many individuals are allergic

FRESH FRUIT BUYING GUIDE

1 lb.	raw amounts	processed yields
apples	3 medium	2 3/4 cups sliced
		1 3/4 cups sauce
apricots	8-12 medium	2 1/2 cups sliced
avocado	2-3 medium	2 1/2 cups sliced
bananas	3-4 medium	2 cups
		1 1/3 cups mashed
blueberries	2 cups	N/A
cantaloupe	1/2 med.	2 cups diced
cherries, sweet unpitted	1 3/4 cups	N/A
cherries, tart pitted	2 1/3 cups	N/A
cranberries	4 cups	4 cups sauce
figs	12 med.	N/A
grapefruit	1 med.	1 cup sections

to sulfites, with reactions ranging from itching and gastrointestinal distress to difficulty in breathing and possibly death.

transitional organic: a claim used to signify food produced in which all conditions for organic certification have been met, except for the required three year length of time for the acreage/product in question to have been free of unapproved inputs or applications.

waxed fruit: fruit coated with a variety of waxes to help prevent moisture loss and reduce wilting and shriveling. Many question whether waxes have been thoroughly researched to be safe for consumption. Fungicides may also be mixed in with the wax.

refrigerate?	storage
yes	2-4 weeks
yes	
when ripe	2-3 days
when ripe	1 week
when ripe	2-3 days
yes	
yes	1 week
when ripe	1 week
yes	2-3 days
yes	2-3 days
yes	1 month
yes	1-2 days
yes	1-2 weeks

FRESH FRUIT BUYING GUIDE

1 lb.	raw amounts	processed yields
grapes, seeded	2 cups	N/A
grapes, seedless	2 1/2 cups	N/A
kiwi	3 med.	1 1/2 cup slices
lemons	4 med.	2/3 cup juice
oranges	2 med.	2 cups sections
		2/3 cup juice
peaches	4 med.	2 cups sliced
pears	4 med.	2 1/8 cups sliced
pineapple	1/2 med.	1 1/2 cups cubed
plums	8-20	2 cups halves
strawberries	2 2/3 cups whole	2 2/3 cups sliced

FRESH, CANNED, FROZEN FRUIT ADDITIVES TO AVOID

added sweeteners (canned and frozen fruit)

artificial colors

irradiation (preservation process labeled with phrase "treated by irradiation" as well as the flower-like international irradiation logo)

pesticides/herbicides (buy organically grown fresh and processed fruits whenever possible)

wax coatings (preservation process used on some apples, avocadoes, grapefruit, lemons, limes, oranges, passion fruit, peaches, pineapples, plums)

refrigerate?	storage
yes	3-5 days
yes	3-5 days
when ripe	1 week
yes	1-2 weeks
yes	1-2 weeks
yes	
when ripe	3-5 days
when ripe	3-5 days
yes	3-5 days
when ripe	3-5 days
yes	3-5 days

HOW TO MINIMIZE EXPOSURE TO PESTICIDE RESIDUES

1. Buy certified organically grown whenever possible.

2. Wash all produce in water before consuming or preparing. A diluted solution of dishwashing soap and water may remove some surface pesticide residues. Systemic pesticides that have been incorporated within the fruit will not be removed.

3. Peel waxed produce. Vegetable wax or food-grade shellacs may be applied to produce to seal in moisture and extend shelf life. It also seals in agricultural chemicals that may have been applied to the produce. Washing will not remove waxes. (By law, grocery stores are required to label produce that has been waxed.) Unfortunately, peeling also reduces the nutrients in the fruit as well as fiber.

PEAK SEASONS FOR FRUIT

Domestically grown produce purchased during its optimum growing season is always the best buy. Locally grown is even better since transportation time to the store is minimal, increasing the likelihood that it is more fresh, retaining more nutrients. Out of season fruits are generally more costly and less flavorful. Imported produce often contains more pesticides than domestically grown produce, possibly pesticides that are banned for use in the United States. Likely, imported produce is also fumigated before it is allowed to enter the country.

The best produce departments will have both the growing method and country of origin clearly displayed for each type of fruit. Only then can you make informed choices.

JANUARY/FEBRUARY

avocado
bananas
bosc pear
comice pear
d'anjou pear
grapefruit
kumquats
kiwi

mandarins
navel oranges
papayas
persimmons
tangerines
temple oranges
valencia oranges
ugli fruit

MARCH, APRIL, MAY

avocado
bananas
berries
blood oranges
d'anjou pear
papayas

pears
pineapple
plums
strawberries
watermelon

JUNE, JULY, AUGUST

apricots
avocado
bananas
bartlett pear
blackberries
blueberries
casaba melons
cantaloupe
cranshaw melons
cherries
figs
grapes
honeydew melons
kiwis
lemons
limes
lychee
mangoes
nectarines
peaches
plums
pineapple
raspberries
watermelons

SEPTEMBER, OCTOBER, NOVEMBER, DECEMBER

apples
avocado
bananas
bartlett pear
bosc pear
casaba melons
coconuts
comice pear
cranberries
d'anjou pear
dates
figs
grapefruit
grapes
honeydew melons
kiwis
kumquats
mandarins
navel oranges
pears
persimmons
plums
pomegranate
prickly pears
quince
Santa Claus melons (Dec.)
temple oranges
ugli fruit

DRIED FRUIT BUYING GUIDE

1 LB.	UNCOOKED	COOKED YIELD
apples	4 1/3 cups	8 cups
apricots	3 cups	4 1/2 cups
bananas	4 1/2 cups	6 cups
cherries	3 1/3 cups	3 1/2 cups
cranberries*	3 2/3 cups	5 cups
currants	3 1/4 cups dry	3 cups cooked
dates, whole	60 small dates	N/A
dates, pitted	2 1/2 cups	N/A
figs	44 small figs	2 2/3 cups chopped
mango	2 1/4 cups	3 cups
papaya	3 1/2 cups	3 1/2 cups
peaches	3 cups	6 cups
pears	26-30 halves	6 1/2 cups
pineapple (diced)	2 cups	2 3/4 cups
prunes, whole	2 1/2 cups	4-4 1/2 cups
prunes, pitted	2 1/4 cups	4-4 1/2 cups
raisins	2 3/4 cups	2 3/4 cups

STORAGE FOR ALL
1 month pantry/6 months fridge

*Dried cranberries are generally sold presweetened.

DRIED FRUIT ADDITIVES TO AVOID

added sugars

partially hydrogenated oil (treated to prolong shelf life and to promote texture and body)

pesticides and herbicides (buy organically grown dried fruit whenever possible)

potassium sorbate (preservative, antimycotic agent)

sodium potassium metabisulfite (preservative, antioxidant, color retention agent)

sulfur dioxide (preservative, antioxidant, color retention agent)

WHY AVOID DRIED DRIED FRUITS TREATED WITH SULFUR DIOXIDE

This additive is known to cause mild to serious reactions in sensitive individuals, with symptoms such as itching, gastrointestinal distress, asthma, difficulty in breathing, wheezing, hives, and, in some cases, death. Since the use of sulfur dioxide is primarily for cosmetic reasons, i.e., to retain bright colors and moist texture, it's an additive that is hard to justify, given its possible effects. Besides, the flavor of dried fruits is even better when they're untreated.

FRUIT JUICE BUYING GUIDE

Choosing the Best Buy for Nutrition
(listed in descending order of nutrient value)

1. freshly extracted juice
2. fresh frozen juice
3. frozen concentrate
4. reconstituted juice
5. canned, bottled, or aseptic-packed juice
6. chilled extracted juice
7. fruit beverages, drinks, spritzers, and cocktails (contain less than 100% juice). These don't even count as a fruit serving.

STORAGE GUIDELINES

TYPE	UNOPENED	AFTER OPENING
freshly extracted	N/A	1-2 days fridge
bottled/canned	1 year shelf	7-10 days fridge
juice boxes	6-9 months shelf	7-10 days fridge
frozen juices (reconstituted)	8-12 months freezer	7-10 days fridge

HEALTHY HINTS

•Look on the label for verification that the juice contains 100% real fruit juice. Fruit beverages, drinks, spritzers, and cocktails contain less than 100% juice.

•Avoid those that list modified juices on the ingredients panel.

•Look on the label to see if all the flavor and body of the juice can actually be attributed to the fruit juice itself. Fruit oils, essences, and pulp added in excess to the amount that would normally be present in the juice or if from a source other than the juice itself must be labeled as separate ingredients on the ingredients panel.

FRESH, CANNED, FROZEN JUICE ADDITIVES TO AVOID

added sugars

artificial color

artificial flavor

artificial sweeteners

brominated vegetable oil (flavor carrier)

modified juices (juices treated to manipulate color, flavor, and aroma)

potassium benzoate (antimycotic agent)

potassium bisulfite (preservative, antioxidant, color retention agent)

potassium metabisulfite (preservative, antioxidant, color retention agent)

potassium sorbate (antimycotic agent)

sodium benzoate (antimycotic agent)

MEAT, POULTRY, FISH, DRY BEANS, EGGS, & NUTS GROUP

WORDS TO KNOW ABOUT MEATS

choice grade: moderately fatty, tender, and flavorful.

cured meats: meats processed with salt, sugar, and often nitrites to preserve meats and impart flavor. Ham, bacon, some sausages, and luncheon meats are cured meats. USDA regulations now mandate a reduction in the amount of nitrite used in cured meats. They also require some form of vitamin C, sodium ascorbate or sodium erythorbate, to scavenge nitrite so less, if any, is available to convert to nitrosamine. Varieties free of sodium nitrite are readily available.

extra lean: contains less than 5 grams total fat, less than 2 grams saturated fat, and less than 95 mg. cholesterol per 3 oz. cooked meat or 2 oz. luncheon meat.

humanely raised: livestock raised in a pasture or low-confinement systems where animals have plenty of room to move and the opportunity to express their normal patterns of behavior.

lean: contains less than 10% total fat, less than 4 grams saturated fat, and less than 95 mg. cholesterol per 3 oz. cooked meat or 2 oz. luncheon meat.

light/lite: contains at least 1/3 fewer calories or 50% less fat than typically found in a particular meat product.

natural meat: The USDA's definition of natural is meat that is minimally processed and free of artificial additives such as preservatives, artificial colors, and artificial flavors. USDA natural cattle are still allowed to be administered antibiotics and growth hormones; however, a withdrawal time is required before slaughter. Nonetheless, many producers and retailers define natural meat as: "raised without antibiotics or growth hormones," signifying the cattle have never received these drugs. Because cattle raised in this manner require a longer maturation time, their meat is typically reported to be more flavorful.

organic meat: meat from animals certified to be raised in accordance with the Federal standards for the organic production of farm animals. Livestock must be fed organically produced feed and raised in a humane manner. Growth promoters and hormones, antibiotics, and synthetic trace elements used to stimulate growth or production are prohibited. Sub-therapeutic doses of antibiotics, synthetic internal parasiticides on a routine basis and medications (other than vaccinations) applied in the absence of illness are also prohibited.

phosphates: additives that help retain moisture during processing and home preparation to make the cured meat more juicy and flavorful. While a small amount may be acceptable, too much means you're paying for water weight rather than meat.

prime grade: the most fatty, tender, and flavorful.

range-fed: livestock grazed on pastureland for most of their lives instead of in a feedlot.

reduced fat: contains at least 25% less fat than typically found in a particular meat product.

select grade: the least fatty, but also less tender and flavorful.

sodium nitrite: an additive use primarily to maintain the pink or red colors in meats and to enhance flavor by inhibiting rancidity. It also protects against bacterial growth. Its use is controversial because when meat containing nitrite is heated at high temperatures, nitrites can combine with protein substances called amines to form nitrosamine, a very potent carcinogenic compound.

HOW MUCH MEAT TO BUY PER PERSON

Boneless cuts (ground meat, boned roasts and steaks, stew meat)	1/4 lb.
Meat with some bone (rib roasts, unboned steaks, chops)	1/3 lb.
Bony cuts (ribs, shanks)	3/4 -1 lb.

TOP LEAN BEEF CUTS
CHOICE OR SELECT GRADE:
top round
eye of round
round tip
sirloin
top loin
tenderloin
bottom round
chuck arm pot roast

PRIME GRADE:
top round
eye of round
round tip

SELECT GRADE:
ribs: small end

TOP LEAN PORK CUTS
tenderloin
center loin
whole ham
boneless ham (regular or extra lean)
Canadian bacon

TOP LEAN LAMB CUTS
CHOICE GRADE:
leg shank
leg sirloin
whole leg
loin
foreshank

FIGURING THE FAT CONTENT OF GROUND BEEF

A more realistic picture of fat content is to translate the percentages of lean to fat by weight into the grams of fat and percentage of total calories from fat you'll actually get from various selections based on a 3 oz. medium broiled portion. Comparable percentage of fat levels in ground pork and lamb will yield similar results.

Sold As	% Calories from Fat	Grams Total Fat
73% lean/27%fat	79%	18 grams
80% lean/20% fat	71%	15 grams
85% lean/15% fat	64%	12 grams
90% lean/10% fat	53%	9 grams
95% lean/5% fat	34%	5 grams

MEAT STORAGE GUIDELINES*

TYPE	REFRIGERATOR	FREEZER
	(36-40° F.)	0° F. or lower
beef cuts	3-4 days	6-12 months
ground beef	1-2 days	3-4 months
lamb cuts	3-5 days	6-9 months
ground lamb	1-2 days	3-4 months
pork cuts	2-3 days	6 months
ground pork	1-2 days	1-3 months
variety meats	1-2 days	3-4 months
leftover cooked meat	3-4 days	2-3 months
luncheon meat	3-5 days	1-2 months
sausage, fresh	2-3 days	1-2 months
sausage, smoked	5-7 days	1-2 months
hot dogs	3-5 days	1-2 months
smoked ham, whole	5-7 days	1-2 months
smoked ham, sliced	3-4 days	1-2 months

*Considering meat may be 1-2 days old in the store. Check for freshness before purchasing.

VEAL

If you insist on eating veal, make sure it is humanely-raised rather than in the manner typically produced in a confined environment that prevents the young calves from manifesting normal behaviors such as eating grasses or grain, turning around, lying down in a natural position, stretching their limbs, and grooming themselves. Since grass and other foods high in iron are not restricted from humanely-raised veal calves, expect the meat to be slightly pink in color.

FRESH, CURED, FROZEN, CANNED MEAT ADDITIVES TO AVOID

artificial color

artificial flavor

BHA (antioxidant, preservative)

BHT (antioxidant, preservative)

livestock raised with antibiotics, hormones, or other drugs

monosodium glutamate (MSG) (flavor enhancer)

sodium nitrite (antioxidant, flavor, color retention agent)

TBHQ (antioxidant, preservative)

FOOD SAFETY TIPS

•Keep meat refrigerated. Be sure the interim time from purchase to home refrigeration is minimal. During hot weather, consider transporting meat in an ice chest.

• Defrost frozen meat only in the refrigerator, not at room temperature or in warm water. Most foodborne pathogens thrive at room temperature.

•You can also thaw meat in a microwave; however, the meat must then be cooked immediately after thawing.

•Be sure to thoroughly wash your hands, kitchen counter top, utensils, dishes, and cutting boards with soap and hot water after contact with raw meat.

•Always marinate meat in the refrigerator. Do not re-use the marinade as a sauce unless it is first brought to a rolling boil.

•Since surface bacteria are transferred to the interior meat during grinding, ground beef should always be cooked medium or well-done, at a temperature of at least 160° F.

•To prevent the possibility of trichinosis, be sure to cook pork to an internal temperature of at least 160° F.

•Do not allow cooked meat to stand at room temperature for more than two hours after cooking. Bacteria thrive at temperatures between 45-115° F., so keep meat either below 40° F. or above 140° F., depending on whether the dish is intended to be served hot or cold.

WORDS TO KNOW ABOUT POULTRY

CHICKEN

breast quarter: includes the wing, breast, and back portion (all white meat).

breast halves or split breast: available with or without the bone, with or without the skin (all white meat).

broiler/fryer: chicken about 7-9 weeks old of either sex, weighing 3-4 1/2 lbs. Broil, fry, roast, steam, or poach.

capon: a castrated male chicken about 4-5 months old, weighing 5-9 lbs. Roast.

drummettes: the first section of a chicken wing, often used for appetizers.

ground chicken: meat from boneless thigh meat, ground with or without the skin (all dark meat).

leg quarters: includes the drumstick, thigh, and back portion (all dark meat).

roaster chicken: about 3-5 months old of either sex, weighing between 4 1/2-8 lbs. Roast.

Rock Cornish hen: 5-6 weeks old of either sex, weighing 1-2 lbs. A cross between the Plymouth Rock chicken and Cornish gamecock, developed to be small but extra meaty. Roast whole or split and grill or broil.

stewing hen: a retired laying hen (female, of course) 10 months of age or older, weighing 3-7 lbs. Cook slowly or stew.

wing: sold with three sections attached, much of which must be discarded yielding little, but delicious, meat (all white meat).

DUCK

broiler/fryer Pekin or Long Island duck: 7-8 weeks old of either sex, weighing less than 3 lbs. Broil or fry.

roaster duck is 8-16 weeks old of either sex, weighing 3-6 lbs. Roast or braise.

extra lean: contains less than 5 grams fat, less than 2 grams saturated fat, and less than 95 mg. cholesterol per 3 oz. cooked poultry or 2 oz. luncheon meat or sausage.

free-range poultry: have access to both an enclosed poultry house that allows over twice the square footage per bird as provided in typical poultry production, as well as an outdoor pen in which to freely roam and forage.

GAME BIRDS

Guinea hen (female): 2-3 lbs. Roast, braise, poach.

Partridge: 1-3 lbs. Young partridge, weighing 1-1 1/2 lbs.—roast or sauté. Older and heavier partridge—braise or stew.

Pheasant: usually farm-raised and sold when 2-4 lbs. Roast or braise.

Quail: about 6-8 oz. Roast, grill, braise, or sauté.

Squab: 4-week-old pigeons of either sex, weighing less than 1 lb. Roast or braise.

GOOSE

mature goose: more than 6 months old of either sex, weighing more than 14 lbs. Braise.

young goose (gosling): less than 6 months old of either sex, weighing between 5-12 lbs. Roast.

housed but uncaged poultry: have access to a roomy poultry house but not to an outdoor pen.

lean: contains less than 10% total fat, less than 4 grams saturated fat, and less than 95 mg. cholesterol per 3 oz. cooked poultry or 2 oz. luncheon meat or sausage.

light/lite: contains at least 1/3 fewer calories or 50% less fat than typically found in a particular poultry product.

naturally raised poultry: raised according to methods that allow for expression of the bird's natural behavior. Check to ensure that no antibiotics have ever been administered.

organically raised: poultry certified to be raised in accordance with the Federal standards for the organic production of farm animals. Livestock must be fed organically produced feed and raised in a humane manner. Growth promoters and hormones, antibiotics and synthetic trace elements used to stimulate growth or production are prohibited. Sub-therapeutic doses of antibiotics, synthetic internal parasiticides on a routine basis and medications (other than vaccinations) applied in the absence of illness are also prohibited.

reduced fat: contains at least 25% less fat than typically found in a particular poultry product.

TURKEY

fryer/roaster: about 10-16 weeks old of either sex, weighing 5-8 lbs. The most tender of turkeys. Roast, broil, grill.

ground turkey: meat from boneless thigh meat, ground with or without the skin (all dark meat).

rolled turkey roast: boned, tied white or combination dark/white turkey meat.

young hen (female) or young tom (male): 4-7 months old, weighing between 8-20 lbs. Roast.

yearling tom: 6-12 month old male turkey, weighing more than 20 lbs. Roast or simmer.

HOW MUCH POULTRY TO BUY PER PERSON

chicken

breast halves	1/2
breast quarters	1
broiler/fryer*, bone-in	3/4-1 lb
bone-less	1/3-1/2 lb.
capon	1/2 lb.
drumsticks	2
ground	1/4 lb.
leg quarters	1
thighs	2
roaster	1/2 lb.
Rock Cornish hen	1 bird
sausage	1/4 lb.
wings	4

* A 3 1/2 lb. whole broiler/fryer chicken with neck and giblets yields slightly over 3 cups of cooked, diced chicken meat without the skin.

turkey

boneless breast	1/3-1/2 lb.
boneless roast	1/3-1/2 lb.
fryer/roaster	3/4-1 lb.
ground	1/4 lb.
hen/tom	1/2-3/4 lb.
sausage	1/4 lb.
thigh (bone-in)	1/2-3/4 lb.
duck/goose	1 lb.

POULTRY STORAGE GUIDELINES*

TYPE	REFRIGERATOR (36-40° F.)	FREEZER (0° F. or lower)
chicken, cut up	1-2 days	9 months
chicken, whole	1-2 days	12 months
chicken giblets	1-2 days	3 months
duck, whole	1-2 days	6 months
goose, whole	1-2 days	6 months
turkey, cut up	1-2 days	6 months
turkey, whole	1-2 days	12 months
cooked poultry**	3-4 days	6 months (covered w/broth) 1 month (no broth)
poultry broth/gravy	1-2 days	2-3 months
cured meats	3-5 days	1-2 months
luncheon meats	3-5 days	1-2 months
hot dogs	3-5 days	1-2 months

*Considering poultry may be 1-2 days old in the store. Check for freshness before purchasing.
**Remove stuffing from cooked poultry. Refrigerate and freeze meat and stuffing separately

FRESH/CURED/FROZEN POULTRY ADDITIVES TO AVOID

artificial colors
artificial flavor
BHA (antioxidant, preservative)
BHT (antioxidant, preservative)
monosodium glutamate (MSG) (flavor enhancer)
partially hydrogenated oil (treated to prolong shelf-
   life and to provide texture and body)
sodium nitrite (antioxidant, flavor, color retention
   agent)

AVOID PATÉS

Avoid goose and duck patés. Both types of birds are
brutally force-fed and confined in small, crowded pens
in order to make their livers unusually large for the
production of paté.

FOOD SAFETY TIPS

•Keep foods refrigerated. Be sure the interim time from
purchase to home refrigeration is minimal and consider transporting them in an ice chest during the hot
weather.

•Thaw frozen poultry only in the refrigerator, never
at room temperature.

REFRIGERATOR THAWING TIMES FOR FROZEN POULTRY

CHICKEN:

less than 4 lbs.	12-24 hours
more than 4 lbs.	1-1 1/2 days

ROCK CORNISH HEN   12 hours

TURKEY:

4-12 lb.	1-2 days
12-20 lb.	2-3 days
20-24 lb.	3-3 1/2 days
halves, quarters, breasts	1-2 days
cut-up pieces	3-9 hours

DUCK, GOOSE: 1-1 1/2 days

•Be sure to thoroughly wash your hands, kitchen counter top, utensils, dishes, and cutting boards with soap and hot water after contact with raw poultry.

•Do not allow cooked poultry to stand at room temperature for more than two hours after cooking. Bacteria thrive at temperatures between 45-115° F., so keep cooked poultry either below 40° F. or above 140° F., depending on whether the dish is intended to be served hot or cold.

•Stuff poultry immediately before roasting, not ahead of time, to prevent bacteria from the raw poultry juices inside the cavity from growing within the stuffing. After cooking, remove the stuffing and serve or refrigerate separately.

WORDS TO KNOW ABOUT FISH/SEAFOOD

aquaculture: the cultivation of seafood in ponds, cages, or pens anchored in natural bodies of water or in man-made tanks supplied with filtered and oxygenated water.

farm-raised fish: another term for aquaculture.

Omega-3 fatty acids: one of two essential fatty acids. This variety, also called alpha-linolenic acid, serves as building blocks for hormone-like compounds (prostaglandins) that influence several important functions within the body.

sulfites/sulfur dioxide: the application of sulfur dioxide, sodium sulfite, sodium and potassium bisulfite, or sodium and potassium metabisulfite to help prevent or bleach out a black pigment on shrimp shells called melanosis or "black spot." Many individuals are allergic to sulfites, with reactions ranging from itching and gastrointestinal distress to difficulty in breathing and possibly death.

surimi: imitation crabmeat, scallops, and lobster made from lean white fish, sugar, sorbitol, salt, water, egg whites, starch, natural and artificial colors, and natural and artificial flavors. Once made into a paste, it is then molded, cooked, and cut into the desired shapes.

HOW TO CHOOSE SAFE SEAFOOD

1. Buy fish only from spotlessly clean, well-maintained markets.
   - Clerks should wear clean aprons, gloves, and hats.
   - Utensils should be immaculate and used only for one particular type of fish, unless washed after each use.
   - Odor within the department should be mildly seaweedy, not a strong, fishy smell.
   - Rather than placed directly on ice, the fish should be in clean metal or plastic containers to protect their texture and appearance and to prevent bacteria contamination.
   - Cooked fish products should be separated from raw.

2. Find out where the fish originated. Buy only fish and seafood harvested as far away as possible from industrial or agricultural areas.

3. Choose fish and seafood free of chemical dips and sulfites used to enhance appearance and color.
   - Whole fish should have eyes that are convex, not sunken, and the skin should be shiny.
   - Fillets should be translucent and light in color, not yellowed or dark. The flesh should be firm and springy when pressed.
   - Clams, mussels, and oysters should be alive with shells that are tightly closed or close upon handling.

4. Buy shellfish only from reputable dealers who buy from harvesters licensed with the National Shellfish Sanitation Program (NSSP).

5. Eat a variety of fish rather than concentrating on one type.

HOW MUCH FISH TO BUY PER PERSON AND APPROPRIATE COOKING METHODS

TYPE	PER PERSON	COOKING METHOD
whole fish (gutted & scaled, fins removed)	12-16 oz.	bake, poach, steam, grill
pan-dressed fish (gutted & scaled, heads, tail, fins removed)	8-12 oz.	bake, pan-fry, oven-fry
steaks crosscut sections of large fish	5-8 oz.	bake, poach, steam, grill, stir-fry strips or cubes
fillets 1/2-1" thick	4-5 oz.	bake, broil, poach, steam, grill, stir-fry strips or cubes
fillets less than 1/2" thick	4-5 oz.	broil, pan-poach, steam, sauté, stir-fry strips

UNDERSTANDING SHRIMP SIZING

Shrimp is sized by the number per pound. Larger sizes are more expensive, worth the price depending on how you plan to serve the fish and on how patient you are with shelling. Nevertheless, after they are cooked and peeled, you'll get the same amount of edible shrimp no matter what size you buy. In general, gauge on buying 1/4 lb. per person. Broil, poach, steam, sauté, boil, stir-fry, grill.

extra colossal	under 10 per pound
colossal	under 15
extra jumbo	16-20
jumbo	21-25
extra large	26-30
large	31-35
medium large	36-40
medium	41-50
small	51-60
extra small	61-70
tiny	over 70

FISH & SEAFOOD STORAGE GUIDELINES

TYPE	REFRIGERATOR (36-40° F.)	FREEZER (0° F. OR LOWER)
fresh lean fillets	1 day	6 months
fresh fatty fillets	1 day	3 months
cooked fish	3 days	3 months
canned fish, opened	3-5 days	3 months in another container
smoked fish, whole	1-2 weeks	not recommended
smoked fish, sliced	3-4 days	not recommended
scallops	1 day	3 months

FISH & SEAFOOD STORAGE GUIDELINES

TYPE	REFRIGERATOR (36-40°F.)	FREEZER (0°F or lower)
shrimp, raw	1-2 days	6 months
shrimp, cooked	3-4 days	2 months
other shellfish	1-2 days	3 months
squid	1 day	3 months
frog legs	1 day	3 months

NUTRITIONAL SUPERSTARS

highest in Omega-3 fatty acids:
sardines
salmon
mackerel
tuna
herring
rainbow trout

lowest in fat
clams
cod
haddock
mahi-mahi
orange roughy
pollock
shrimp
sole
flounder
Pacific rockfish
whiting

FISH/SEAFOOD ADDITIVES TO AVOID

artificial colors
artificial flavors
chlorine dips (preservative)
monosodium glutamate (MSG) (flavor enhancer)
partially hydrogenated oil (treated to prolong shelf
  life and to provide texture and body)
sodium & potassium bisulfite (preservative,
  antioxidant, color retention agent)
sodium potassium metabisulfite (preservative,
  antioxidant, color retention agent)

sodium sulfite (preservative, antioxidant, color retention agent)

sulfur dioxide (preservative, antioxidant, color retention agent)

TBHQ (antioxidant, preservative)

FOOD SAFETY TIPS

•Keep fish refrigerated. Be sure the interim time from purchase to home refrigeration is minimal. Consider transporting them in an ice chest during hot weather.

•Thaw frozen fish only in the refrigerator, NOT AT ROOM TEMPERATURE.

•Allow about 24 hours for a 1 lb. package. To retain more juices and moisture, do not thaw frozen fish completely. If a quick thaw is needed, place the fish in a "zipper-lock" type plastic bag and place in a pan of cold water in the refrigerator.

•Use thawed frozen fish within 24 hours.

•Be sure to thoroughly wash your hands, kitchen counter top, utensils, dishes, and cutting boards with soap and hot water after contact with raw fish and seafood.

•Do not allow cooked fish to stand at room temperature for more than two hours after cooking. Bacteria thrive at temperatures between 45-115° F., so keep fish either below 40° F. or above 140° F., depending on whether the dish is intended to be served hot or cold.

WORDS TO KNOW ABOUT BEANS

heirloom beans: old-fashioned varieties of beans that are regaining popularity due to their remarkable flavors and nutritional attributes.

hybrid beans: varieties of beans specially developed for a number of reasons: to resist fungi and insect infestations, for improved digestibility, and for their beauty, flavor, and texture.

miso: a fermented soybean paste made by mixing cooked soybeans or chickpeas with koji (grain inoculated with Aspergillus orzae), salt, water, and, in some varieties, grain. Depending on the type of miso, the mixture is then fermented from 2 months to 3 years. It can be used in soups or sauces instead of bouillon or as a base for stews, gravies, salad dressings, dips, or spreads.

organically grown: certified to be produced according to the requirements of the Federal organic certification program using management-intensive methods designed to promote and enhance soil-fertility, biological cycles, and biodiversity. No prohibited fertilizers, chemical pesticides, herbicides, or fungicides may have been applied for at least 3 years prior to marketing as organic.

Organic foods are processed, packaged, transported, and stored to retain maximum nutritional value, without the use of artificial preservatives or colorings, irradiation, or toxic synthetic chemicals.

silken tofu: a type of tofu popular in traditional Japanese cuisine that is much lighter, more delicate, and sweeter-tasting than regular tofu. As it resembles a custard or thick cream, it can be used to impart a creamy texture to soups, shakes, dips, dressings, and sauces. Silken tofu is often sold in aseptic, shelf-stable containers.

tempeh: a traditional Indonesian soy food made by culturing cooked, cracked soybeans and often a grain with a starter called Rhizopus oligosporus. After an incubation period of 24 hours, the soybeans form into a cake. Its chewy texture and mild, mushroomy flavor make it an excellent meat substitute.

tofu: a traditional Oriental soy food made by coagulating soymilk obtained from grinding and cooking soybeans and pressing the curds into blocks. Its soft, custard-like consistency and relatively bland flavor make tofu a very versatile, high-protein food ready to be seasoned or cooked in a myriad of ways. It is also frequently used as a dairy substitute for dips and dressings.

TVP™: the abbreviation for texturized vegetable protein. It is made by removing 90% of the soluble sugars from defatted soy flour. The resulting concentrated protein is then extruded into granules and chunks. Rehydrated TVP™ has the appearance and texture of meat.

BEANS BUYING GUIDE

Select beans with smooth surfaces and bright colors. Beans that are too old or too dry will have cracked seams or dull, wrinkled

I lb.	UNCOOKED	COOKED YIELDS
adzuki beans	2 1/4 cups	5 cups
anasazi beans	2 1/2 cups	5-6 cups
black beans	2 1/2 cups	5-6 cups
black-eyed peas	2 1/2 cups	5-6 cups
garbanzo beans	2 1/2 cups	5 cups
great northerns	2 1/2 cups	5-6 cups
kidney beans	2 1/2 cups	5-6 cups
lentils, green	2 1/2 cups	5 cups
lentils, red	2 1/2 cups	5 cups
lima beans	2 1/2 cups	5 1/2 cups
mung beans	2 1/2 cups	5 cups
navy beans	2 1/3 cups	5 1/2 cups

Note: Cooked beans can store for up to 5 days in fridge or 6 months in the freezer.

surfaces. Avoid buying beans that contain too many splits.

STORAGE/COOKING

3-12 months in cool area
1 1/2 hours simmer; 25 min. pressure cook

3-12 months in cool area
1 1/2 hours simmer; 25 min. pressure cook

3-12 months in cool area
1 1/2 hours simmer; 25 min. pressure cook

3-12 months in cool area
1 1/4 hours simmer; 25 min. pressure cook

3-12 months in cool area
2 1/2 hours simmer; 30 min. pressure cook

3-12 months in cool area
1 1/2 hours simmer; 25 min. pressure cook

3-12 months in cool area
1 1/2 hours simmer; 25 min. pressure cook

3-12 months in cool area
45 minutes simmer; 25 min. pressure cook

3-12 months in cool area
25 minutes simmer; don't pressure cook

3-12 months in cool area
1 1/2 hours simmer; don't pressure cook

3-12 months in cool area
1 1/4 hours simmer; 25 min. pressure

3-12 months in cool area
2 hours simmer; 25 min. pressure

*See package for freshness dating. Various packing methods yield a variance in refrigerator life. Once tofu is removed from its packaging, it must be stored in water which is refreshed daily.

I lb.	UNCOOKED	COOKED YIELDS
pinto beans	2 1/2 cups	5-6 cups
red beans	2 1/2 cups	5-6 cups
soybeans	2 3/4 cups	5-6 cups
split peas	2 1/4 cups	5 cups
tempeh (8 oz.)	1 1/3 cups	1 1/3 cups
tofu, firm (16 oz.)	3 cups cubed	3 cups cubed
	2 cups mashed or puréed	
tofu, silken (10 oz.)	1 cup mashed	

TIPS FOR OPTIMUM DIGESTION

1. Soak the beans and discard the soaking water prior to cooking.

2. Cook beans with bay leaf, cumin, or epazote.

3. Cook the beans thoroughly.

4. Avoid beans cooked with sweeteners.

5. Eat smaller quantities until your body adjusts to digesting them.

6. Focus on legumes that are easier to digest: anasazi beans, adzuki beans, black-eyed peas, lentils, mung beans, tofu, and tempeh.

7. Sprinkle a few drops of BEANO™ on your beans or ingest 2-3 BEANO™ tablets to supply a natural digestive enzyme.

STORAGE/COOKING*

3-12 months in cool area, 2 hours simmer; 25 min. pressure

3-12 months in cool area, 1 1/2 hours simmer; 25 min. pressure

3-12 months in cool area, 3-4 hours simmer; 1 1/2 hours pressure cook

3-12 months in cool area, 1 1/4 hours simmer; 25 min. pressure

7 days in fridge, 6 months in freezer

7 days in fridge,* 6 months in freezer

Aseptic packed: 9 months on shelf. Refrigerate when open. Don't freeze.

BEAN ADDITIVES TO AVOID

canned varieties (as found in pre-cooked bean products):
artificial flavors
calcium disodium EDTA (antioxidant, sequestrant)
disodium EDTA (antioxidant, sequestrant)
excess sodium
lard (high in saturated fat)
monosodium glutamate (MSG) (flavor enhancer)
partially hydrogenated oil (treated to prolong shelf
    life and to promote texture and body)
potassium sorbate (preservative, antimycotic agent)
sodium nitrite (antioxidant, flavor, color retention
    agent)

WORDS TO KNOW ABOUT EGGS

egg substitutes: alternatives to eggs used by individuals who desire the cooking properties or flavor of eggs but are concerned about the amount of cholesterol found in each egg. Commercial varieties are available in two basic models. Most familiar are the liquid substitutes based primarily on pasteurized egg whites mixed with oil, cornstarch, emulsifiers, and, in some brands, artificial coloring. Another type of egg substitute is made by first treating the egg yolk to remove much of the cholesterol and then recombining it with the egg white to produce a pasteurized liquid whole egg product. Commercial vegetarian versions are made from potato starch, tapioca flour, leavening agents, and a vegetable-derived gum.

fertile eggs: produced by hens who have mated with a rooster. Hens are allowed to freely roam and express their natural behaviors at least within a chicken house and, in some cases, a yard. In addition to supporting a more humane environment for hens, many people claim fertile eggs taste better than eggs from standard caged hens. The higher price of fertile eggs is generally attributed to higher production costs.

graded eggs: inspected by a USDA inspector according to the interior quality of the egg and the condition and appearance of the shell at the time the egg is packed.

Grade AA: tops in quality and freshness. Yolk is firmly centered, white is clear, firm, and thick, and the overall height of the egg is high. Best for poaching, frying, and cooking in the shell when the appearance of the egg is important.

Grade A: Not as satisfactory for poaching but still excellent for frying and cooking purposes. Grade A eggs may be up to 30 days old.

Grade B: Can be used when the appearance of the egg doesn't matter, i.e. scrambled eggs or blended cooked foods. Shells may be slightly abnormal in shape.

salmonella: a term used to describe a group of related bacteria that cause symptoms similar to the intestinal flu. Most egg-related cases of salmonella food poisoning have occurred from using cracked or leaking eggs or from eating raw or undercooked eggs.

standard hatchery eggs: nonfertile, mass-produced eggs laid by hens confined 3-5 per small cage with little room for movement.

yard eggs: produced from free-range hens allowed to express their natural behaviors within a chicken house as well as a yard. Yard eggs are not necessarily fertile.

BROWN VS. WHITE EGGS
The color of the eggshell indicates only that a certain variety of hen laid the egg. Both brown and white eggs are equal nutritionally.

EGG SIZING COMPARISON CHART

Determined according to the minimum weight per dozen. Most recipes are based on large eggs but other sizes can be substituted. Use the following chart as a guide when substituting other sizes of eggs for large eggs.

Large	Jumbo	X-Large	Medium	Small
1 egg	1	1	1	1
2 eggs	2	2	2	3
3 eggs	2	3	3	4
4 eggs	3	4	5	5
5 eggs	4	4	6	7
6 eggs	5	5	7	8

EGG STORAGE GUIDELINES

TYPE	REFRIGERATION
fresh, whole	3-4 weeks
egg yolks	1-2 days
egg whites	3-4 days
hard cooked, unpeeled*	5-7 days
hard cooked, peeled*	4-5 days

*Eggs that are 2 weeks old are best for hard-boiling since they peel more easily.

EGG ADDITIVES TO AVOID

(as found in egg sustitutes)
artificial colors
artificial flavors
potassium sorbate (preservative, antimycotic agent)

FOOD SAFETY TIPS

•Never use cracked or leaking eggs.

•Keep raw and cooked eggs refrigerated at temperatures below 40° F.

•Avoid beverages and foods made with raw eggs that do not undergo further cooking.

•Cook eggs thoroughly:

scrambled	at least 1 minute
sunnyside up	5 minutes
fried over easy	3 minutes on the first side and 2 minutes on second
poached	5 minutes
boiled eggs	7 minutes
meringue-topped pies	25-27 minutes baked in 325° F. oven

•Refrigerate cooked eggs and egg dishes quickly. Never consume eggs and egg dishes left unrefrigerated for more than 2 hours.

AVOIDING SALMONELLA FOOD POISONING

Salmonella bacteria, the most commonly reported source of foodborne illness, is caused by eating raw or undercooked foods such as eggs, poultry, meats, and dairy products.

Symptoms of salmonella food poisoning (headache, abdominal pain, diarrhea, fever, and nausea) generally begin 12-48 hours after eating the contaminated food.

As with poultry and meats, thorough cooking of eggs is the best way to avoid salmonellosis (see above timing chart listed in Food Safety Tips). Although this would seem to preclude the preparation and consumption of foods and drinks that are traditionally made with raw eggs such as Caesar salad, hollandaise sauce, home-made mayonnaise, homemade ice cream, and egg nog, the use of pasteurized eggs, sold in some grocery stores, makes these foods safe to eat.

If you have difficulty finding them, low-cholesterol egg-based egg substitutes are the next best solution. They are suitable for any recipe calling for unseparated eggs, including recipes that depend on the addition of raw, uncooked eggs.

WORDS TO KNOW ABOUT NUTS AND SEEDS

aflatoxin: a carcinogenic toxin produced by a fungus, Aspergillus flavus, that can grow on grains, nuts, and peanuts.. It produces best on plants that are weakened by insects or stressed from the lack of moisture during a drought.

gomasio: a low-sodium condiment made by roasting and grinding sesame seeds with salt in a proportion of about 14 to 1.

mechanically hulled: sesame seeds that are hulled in a chemical-free manner. The seeds are first steam-heated to loosen the hulls and then mechanically rolled to remove the hulls. Mechanically hulled sesame seeds have a dull, off-white appearance with some color variation.

nut milks: a nondairy milk substitute made by blending ground nuts with water and an emulsifier like flaxseeds or lecithin and then straining away the solids.

organically grown: certified to be produced according to the requirements of the Federal organic certification program using management-intensive methods designed to promote and enhance soil fertility, biological cycles, and biodiversity. No prohibited fertilizers, chemical pesticides, herbicides, or fungicides may have been applied for at least 3 years prior to marketing as organic.

Foods labeled as organic are processed, packaged, transported, and stored to retain maximum nutritional value, without the use of artificial preservatives or colorings, irradiation, or toxic synthetic chemicals.

sesame butter: a peanut butter-like spread made from whole ground sesame seeds. Darker in color and stronger in flavor than tahini, sesame butter is used primarily as a spread rather than as an ingredient in cooking.

tahini: a creamy peanut butter-like spread made from hulled sesame seeds. Tahini made from raw sesame seeds has a nutty, subtly sweet flavor and thin consistency. In contrast, tahini made from roasted sesame seeds has a deeper, richer flavor. Tahini can be used as a spread or as a creamy addition to soups, dressings, dips, and sauces.

tamari roasted nuts/seeds: nuts or seeds roasted with a sprinkling of naturally produced soy sauce, giving them a rich, salty flavor.

NUTS/SEEDS BUYING AND STORAGE GUIDE

Avoid nuts that are moldy, discolored, or shriveled. The insides of a split nut/seed should be of uniform color. Various shades of darkness inside indicates rancidity. Buy bulk nuts only from stores that sell them from clean containers in a clean area and rotate their stock frequently. Otherwise, packaged nuts may be a better alternative. Stores with infrequent sales of nuts should refrigerate their stock.

1 LB. NUTS	CUP YIELD	REFRIGERATOR	FREEZER
almonds (in shell)	1 1/4 cups (shelled)	12 months	12 months
almonds, shelled	3 cups	6 months	9 months
brazil nuts	3 1/4 cups	3-6 months	9 months
cashews	3 1/4 cups	3-6 months	9 months
chestnuts (in shell)	2 1/2 cups (shelled)	4-6 months	9-12 months shelled & blanched
coconut (dried)	5 3/4 cups	1 month	6 months
flaxseeds	2 2/3 cups	6 months	12 months
hazelnuts (in shell)	1 1/2 cups (shelled)	9 months	12 months
hazelnuts, shelled	3 1/2 cups	3-6 months	9 months
macadamia	3 1/3 cups	3-6 months	9 months
peanuts (in shell)	2 1/3 cups (shelled)	6 months	9-12 months
peanuts, shelled	3 cups	3 months	6 months
pecans (in shell)	2 cups (shelled)	6 months	12 months
pecans, shelled	4 cups	3 months	12 months
pine nuts	3 cups	1 month	6 months
pistachios (in shell)	3 1/2-4 cups	3 months	12 months
pumpkin seeds	7 cups	6 months	12 months
sesame seeds, whole	3 1/8 cups	6 months	12 months
sesame seeds, hulled	3 1/2 cups	6 months	12 months
sunflower seeds (in shell)	2 1/2 cups	12 months	12 months
sunflower seeds, shelled	3 1/4 cups	6 months	12 months
walnuts (in shell)	2 cups	6 months	12 months
walnuts, shelled	3 1/2 cups	3 months	12 months

Note: Nuts in shell can also be stored in a cool, dry place for an average of 2-3 months. Nut milks will keep up to 5-7 days in the refrigerator. Suggested storage times listed above are based on the use of very fresh nuts and seeds.

NUTS NUTRITION

VARIETY	% CALORIES FROM FAT	PREDOMINANT TYPE OF FAT
chestnuts	13%	monounsaturated
flaxseed	64%	superunsaturated (Omega-3)
cashews	72%	monounsaturated
pumpkin seeds	76%	polyunsaturated
sesame seeds	76%	mono/polyunsaturated
peanuts	77%	monounsaturated
pistachios	78%	monounsaturated
sunflower seeds	78%	polyunsaturated
almonds	81%	monounsaturated
pine nuts	86%	polyunsaturated
pecans	87%	monounsaturated
coconut	88%	saturated
walnuts	89%	polyunsaturated
brazil nuts	92%	polyunsaturated
hazelnuts	92%	monounsaturated
macadamia nuts	95%	monounsaturated

NUT BUTTERS BUYING GUIDE

Buy organically grown whenever possible to avoid pesticides (often concentrated in the fat of a plant) and increased likelihood of aflatoxins. Unsalted nut butters are a better nutritional choice than salted varieties.

similar in fat content

cashew butter	often contains added oil, raising cashew's fat content to more nearly equal peanut and sesame butters. Use as a spread or dilute to make creamy sauces.

peanut butter	valencia peanuts yield best flavor. Available smooth and crunchy.
sesame butter	ground from whole sesame = hearty flavor, thicker texture for use as a spread.
sesame tahini	ground from hulled sesame = lighter flavor, thinner texture for dressings, spreads, sauces.

higher in fat

almond butter	Available smooth and crunchy. A delicious alternative to peanut butter.

highest in fat

hazelnut butter	Use as a spread, dilute for a sauce, and add to baked goods.

NUT BUTTER STORAGE GUIDELINES

unopened: 12 months unrefrigerated in cool, dry
    conditions
opened: 2-3 months in refrigerator

NUTS/NUT BUTTER/NUT MIXES ADDITIVES TO AVOID

added sugars
artificial color
artificial flavor
disodium guanylate (flavor enhancer)
disodium inosinate (flavor enhancer)
hydrogenated oil (treated to prolong shelf life and to
    provide texture and body)
monosodium glutamate (MSG) (flavor enhancer)
sulfur dioxide (preservative, antioxidant, color
    retention agent)
TBHQ (antioxidant, preservative)

WORDS TO KNOW ABOUT DAIRY PRODUCTS

acidophilus: often dubbed "friendly bacteria." Dairy products that contain Lactobacillus acidophilus are often recommended as a way to reintroduce beneficial bacteria to the colon after bouts of diarrhea or after using antibiotics.

bovine somatotropin (BST): a bioengineered growth hormone developed to increase milk production from cows, despite the fact that there is already a glut of milk in the United States and that the drug undermines the health of the cow. BST-treated cows have higher levels of mastitis (infections of the udder), a condition that is treated with antibiotics or other drugs. Unfortunately, it is difficult to know which brands to avoid since manufacturers who previously labeled their products "free of BST" were sued by the manufacturer of the drug and warned by the FDA that their statements alluding to the fact that milk from cows treated with BST was inferior were false and misleading. Your safest bet is to buy organically produced milk which is required to be produced without drugs, including BST.

homogenization: distributes fat particles evenly throughout the milk so there is no separation of the cream from the rest of the milk.

kefir: a thick beverage with a flavor and texture similar to a tangy milkshake. It is made by incubating naturally formed organisms made of milk proteins overnight in milk. It is sold both plain and fruit-flavored.

lactase-treated milk: milk to which lactase, an enzyme that breaks down lactose, is added. Individuals who are allergic to lactose can drink lactase-treated milk or add lactase tablets to milk.

lactose intolerance: the inability to metabolize some or all lactose (the primary carbohydrate in milk) into glucose, the usable form of sugar the body requires for energy. Symptoms arise from digestive-tract distress, including cramps, flatulence, and/or diarrhea.

organic dairy products: verified to be produced according to the requirements of the Federal organic certification program. Livestock must be fed organically produced feed and raised in a humane manner, including pasturing, free stalls, and comfortable bedding. Growth promoters and hormones, antibiotics and synthetic trace elements used to stimulate growth or production are prohibited. Sub-therapeutic doses of antibiotics, synthetic internal parasiticides on a routine basis and medications (other than vaccinations) applied in the absence of illness are also prohibited. All processing of organic dairy products must be entirely separate from nonorganic products.

pasteurization: a method in which milk is heated to 161° F. for 15 seconds to kill yeasts, mold, pathogenic microorganisms, and most of the less harmful strains of bacteria.

pasteurized processed cheese food is made by combining pasteurized processed cheese with whey, cream, milk, nonfat dry milk, or buttermilk. Artificial colors and flavorings may also be included.

pasteurized processed cheeses are made by mixing several aged and unaged natural cheeses with an emulsifier to make a smooth, homogeneous mixture. Pasteurization of the cheese effectively stops the aging process, but because it does not kill all bacteria, preservatives and a great deal of salt may be added to improve shelf life.

quarg: a soft, white, lowfat cheese with a slightly acidic taste and smooth, spreadable texture. It can be used as a substitute for sour cream, cream cheese, ricotta, and cottage cheese.

raw milk cheese: cheese made from unpasteurized milk required to be aged at least 60 days before sale to ensure any harmful bacteria is eliminated by the naturally occurring acidity of the cheese. Cheese aficionados claim raw milk cheese tastes better than cheese from pasteurized milk.

rennet: a preparation made from an enzyme extracted from the lining of calves' stomachs to separate the curds from the whey when making cheese.

rennetless: a nonanimal-based alternative to rennet made from an enzyme produced from a mold culture or from bioengineered bacteria

ultrapasteurization: a method in which milk is heated to 280° F. for 2-4 seconds to kill more bacteria than pasteurization. Used frequently for whipping cream and half & half products since it significantly extends shelf life.

FRESH & CULTURED DAIRY PRODUCTS BUYING GUIDE

TYPE	YIELD	STORAGE
8 oz. cottage cheese	1 cup	1 week in fridge, see dating
1/2 pint fresh cream	1 cup	1-4 days in fridge, 4 months in freezer
1/2 pint sour cream	1 cup	1-3 weeks in fridge, don't freeze
1/2 pint ultrapasteurized cream	1 cup	2-4 weeks in fridge, 4 months in freezer
1/2 pint whipped cream	1 cup unwhipped	2-4 weeks in fridge, don't freeze. Homemade whipped cream lasts 1 day

FRESH & CULTURED DAIRY PRODUCTS BUYING GUIDE

TYPE	YIELD	STORAGE
1 quart fresh milk	4 cups	1-5 days in fridge, 3 months in freezer
1-1 1/3 cups dry milk	1 quart reconstituted	3 months in cool, dry area, 6 months in freezer
1 lb. nonfat dry milk	3 2/3 cups dry	see above
1 pint yogurt	2 cups	1-3 weeks in fridge, 1 1/2 months in freezer

FAT COMPARISON

1 CUP SERVING	FAT	CHOLESTEROL	% CALORIES FROM FAT
whole milk	8 grams	33 mg	48%
2% milk	5 grams	22 mg.	37%
skim milk	trace	4 mg.	5%
goat milk	10 grams	28 mg.	54%
buttermilk	2 grams	9 mg.	2%
whole yogurt	7.4 grams	29 mg.	48%
lowfat yogurt	3.5 grams	14 mg	21%
nonfat yogurt	trace	4 mg.	3%
frozen yogurt	3 grams	10 mg.	10%
ice cream, premium	24 grams	90 mg.	61%
ice cream, regular	14 grams	60 mg.	54%
ice milk	6 grams	20 mg.	28%

FRESH/CULTURED/FROZEN DAIRY ADDITIVES TO AVOID

artificial sweeteners

artificial colors

artificial flavors

carbomethylcellulose (thickener, binder, stabilizer)

milk from cows administered synthetic BST (bovine somatotropin)

potassium sorbate (preservative, antimycotic agent)

sodium benzoate (preservative, antimycotic agent)

CHEESE BUYING GUIDE

TYPE	CUP YIELD
8 oz. cream cheese	1 cup
1 lb. hard cheeses	4 cups grated
1 lb. semi-firm cheeses	5 cups grated
1/4 lb. Parmesan or romano	1 1/4 cups grated

CHEESE STORAGE GUIDELINES

TYPE	REFRIGERATOR	FREEZER
Fresh Cheeses		
Chevre	7-10 days	not recommended
Cream Cheese	1-2 weeks	not recommended
Farmer's Cheese	1-2 weeks	6 months
Fresh Mozzarella	2-3 days	not recommended
Kefir Cheese	1-2 weeks	not recommended
Ricotta	1-2 weeks	6 months

CHEESE STORAGE GUIDELINES

TYPE	REFRIGERATOR	FREEZER
Soft cheeses		
Brie	3-5 days	6 months
Camembert	3-5 days	6 months
Muenster	2-4 weeks	6 months
Port du Salut	2-4 weeks	6 months
Washed rind cheeses		
Appenzeller	4 weeks	6 months
Brick	4-8 weeks	6 months
Limburger	1-2 weeks	6 months
Blue cheeses		
Danish Blue	2-4 weeks	6 months
Gorgonzola	2-4 weeks	6 months
Roquefort	2-4 weeks	6 months
Stilton	2-4 weeks	6 months
Maytag blue	2-4 weeks	6 months
Shropshire Blue	2-4 weeks	6 months
Semi-firm cheeses		
Bel Paese	3-4 weeks	6 months
Colby	4-8 weeks	6 months
Edam	4-8 weeks	6 months
Gouda	4-8 weeks	6 months
Havarti	3-4 weeks	6 months
Monterey Jack	2-4 weeks	6 months
Mozzarella	2-4 weeks	6 months
Provolone	8-12 weeks	6 months
Tilsit	2-4 weeks	6 months
Firm or hard cheeses		
Cheddars	4-8 weeks	6 months
Cheddar, goat	4-8 weeks	6 months
Double Gloucester	4-8 weeks	6 months

TYPE	REFRIGERATOR	FREEZER
Emmenthaler	4 weeks	6 months
English Cheshire	4-8 weeks	6 months
Feta	8-12 weeks	not recommended
Gruyere	4 weeks	6 months
Jarlsberg	4 weeks	6 months
Sage Derby	4-8 weeks	6 months
Swiss	4 weeks	6 months
GRATING		
Asiago	2-6 months	6 months
Parmesan	9-12 months	not needed
Pecorino Romano	9-12 months	not needed

Note: wrap cheese in foil or plastic wrap to keep it from drying out and from picking up unwanted moisture and odors from other foods.

Cheeses that are frozen will have a crumbly texture when thawed. For best flavor and texture, just buy the amount of cheese you can use within the recommended refrigerated shelf-life guidelines.

CHEESES LOWEST IN FAT

Cheese's flavor and texture comes mostly from fat. To include cheese in a well-balanced diet it is best to use it sparingly as a condiment, not as a focal point. The following cheeses are specially made to be lower in fat, based on lowfat milk or, as Parmesan, are typically sprinkled lightly over foods, approximately 2 TB. per serving.

Cabot VitaLait™ Cheddar
Fromage Blanc
Gouda light
Havarti light
Jarlsberg light
Lappi

Mozzarella, part-skim
Neufchatel
Parmesan
Quarg
Swiss light
Yogurt Cheese

CHEESE ADDITIVES TO AVOID

artificial colors

milk from cows administered synthetic BST (bovine
    somatotropin)

potassium sorbate (preservative, antimycotic agent)

sorbic acid (preservative, antimycotic agent)

NONDAIRY ALTERNATIVES

milk: soy milk, nut milk, rice milk, amasake

cheese: soy cheese*, almond "cheez"*

frozen treats: soy-based ice creams, rice-based frozen
    desserts, fruit sorbet

yogurt: soy yogurt, homemade nut milk yogurt

*Contains sodium caseinate, a milk protein, as a
binder. If you're sensitive/allergic to milk protein, you
should avoid these cheese substitutes. If you're sensi-
tive/allergic to lactose but not to milk protein, these
may be well tolerated. (Anyone with a severe milk al-
lergy should check with his/her doctor before experi-
menting with nondairy cheese substitutes.)

NONDAIRY ADDITIVES TO AVOID

artificial color

partially hydrogenated oil (treated to prolong shelf-
    life and to provide texture and body)

sodium stearoyl lactylate (emulsifer, whipping agent)

WORDS TO KNOW ABOUT FATS AND OILS

cholesterol: A waxy substance made primarily in the liver and in cells lining the small intestine, is an essential constituent of cell membranes and nerve fibers, and a building block of certain hormones. Too high a level of serum cholesterol has been linked to coronary heart disease and stroke.

clarified butter: also known as ghee. Butter from which the water and milk solids have been removed, leaving pure golden butter fat. Clarified butter will not scorch or turn black when heated to frying or sautéing temperatures.

fat-free: contains less than 0.5 grams of fat per standard serving size.

ghee: see clarified butter

high density lipoproteins (HDL): Also known as "good" cholesterol, HDL lipoproteins pick up the cholesterol deposits and bring them to the liver for recycling or disposal. A higher proportion of HDL lipoproteins to LDL lipoproteins represents more active cholesterol, a lower risk of developing atherosclerosis, and a lower risk of heart attack and stroke.

hydrogenation: a chemical process that transforms liquid vegetable oils into margarine and shortenings that are solid or semisolid at room temperature. Manufacturers like hydrogenated fats because they are cheap, emulate the consistency and "mouthfeel" of butter and lard, and are more resistant to rancidity so shelf life can be extended much beyond normal expectancy. (See trans-fatty acids, p.118.)

low density lipoproteins (LDL): These are the lipoproteins that have become known as "bad" cholesterol because after they deliver the cholesterol actually needed by the cells, they deposit any excess in arterial walls and other tissues.

low fat: contains 3 grams or less fat per standard serving size.

mechanically pressed oil: also known as expeller pressing (and sometimes "cold-pressed"), extracts oil through the use of continuously driven screws that crush the seed or other oil-bearing material into a pulp from which the oil is expressed. Mechanically pressed oil can then be refined or left unrefined.

monounsaturated fat: The substitution of monounsaturated fats for some saturated fats may help reduce total blood cholesterol and LDL cholesterol while preserving the beneficial HDL cholesterol that helps eliminate excess cholesterol.

Omega-3 fatty acid: It is one of the essential fatty acids that must be obtained from food for cell membrane integrity, energy production, growth, immune response, and reproduction.

organic: oil verified to be grown and produced according to the requirements of the Federal organic certification program using management-intensive methods designed to promote and enhance soil fertility, biological cycles, and biodiversity. No prohibited fertilizers, chemical pesticides, herbicides, or fungicides may have been applied for at least 3 years prior to marketing as organic. Foods sold as organic are processed, packaged, transported, and stored to retain maximum nutritional value, without the use of artificial preservatives or colorings, irradiation, or toxic synthetic chemicals.

polyunsaturated fat: the substitution of polyunsaturated fats for some saturated fats tends to decrease total blood cholesterol, at the same time it also reduces the effect of the beneficial HDL cholesterol.

reduced fat: contains at least 25% less fat per standard serving size than what is typically found within the particular product being compared.

refined oils: processed to remove all the bioactive components found in unrefined oil that make it more prone to oxidation. While extensive processing significantly reduces their nutritive content (the oil's essential fatty acids remain) and makes them bland in flavor, aroma, and color, they are much more chemically stable, making them suitable for high-heat cooking.

saturated fat: High intakes of saturated fats are associated with elevated risks of coronary heart disease, obesity, and cancers of the colon, prostate, and breast.

solvent-extracted oil: uses hexane, a highly flammable, colorless, volatile solvent to extract the maximum amount of oil from the seed or oil-bearing material. Although much of the hexane may be removed when the oil/solvent blend is heated and then distilled, many people question the use of a known carcinogen in the processing of food when a nonchemical mechanical-pressing alternative is readily available.

trans-fatty acids: a type of fatty acid formed in the process of hydrogenation in which one of the existing hydrogens at the normal flexible carbon double bond in the fat molecule flips and rotates, make a more rigid molecule that the body does not metabolize in the body. Deformed cellular structures may result, increasing cancer risks, accelerated aging and degenerative changes in tissues, and the potential for heart disease.

unrefined oils: minimally processed to retain most of the nutrients originally found in the natural oil, including vitamin E, carotenes (vitamin A precursors), chlorophyll, phytosterols, and phospholipids, most notably lecithin. These and other biochemical compounds in the oil also provide unrefined oil's characteristic full-bodied flavor, enticing aroma, and deep, rich color. Since unrefined oils are more sensitive to heat and light, they should be used at temperatures no higher than 350° F.

BUYING BUTTER OR MARGARINE

Butter: salted vs. unsalted: Salted butter keeps longer but is more likely to stick to pans and skillets. Unsalted butter, also called sweet butter, has a more delicate flavor. Since it doesn't keep as long, it requires the use of very fresh cream by the manufacturer.

Margarines: If you insist on using a hydrogenated fat like margarine, minimize your intake of trans-fatty acids by choosing soft tub-like or liquid "squeeze" margarines instead of the more hydrogenated stick versions. The first ingredient listed on the label should be a liquid vegetable oil rather than partially hydrogenated fat.

FAT, OIL, MARGARINE ADDITIVES TO AVOID

artificial color

artificial flavor

BHT/BHA (antioxidant, preservative)

calcium disodium EDTA (antioxidant, sequestrant)

caprenin (fat substitute)

fat substitutes except vegetable gums, hydrolyzed oat flour, malto-dextrins

hydrogenated fats (treated to prolong shelf life and to provide texture and body)

partially hydrogenated fats (treated to prolong shelf life and to provide texture and body)

potassium sorbate (preservative, antimycotic agent)

sodium benzoate (preservative, antimycotic agent)

SALAD DRESSING ADDITIVES TO AVOID

artificial color

artificial flavor

calcium disodium EDTA (antioxidant, sequestrant)

disodium guanylate (flavor enhancer)

disodium inosinate (flavor enhancer)

OILS AT A GLANCE

OIL	PROCESS-ING	PRIMARY FATTY ACID	FLAVOR
almond	refined	monounsaturated	mildly sweet & nutty
avocado	refined	monounsaturated	nutty, sharp
canola	refined	monounsaturated + 10% Omega-3 fatty acids	mildly nutty
coconut oil	refined	saturated	nutty
corn	unrefined	polyunsaturated	buttery
corn	refined	polyunsaturated	buttery
cottonseed	refined	polyunsaturated	bland

monosodium glutamate (MSG) (flavor enhancer)
potassium sorbate (preservative, antimycotic agent)
sulfiting agents (preservative, antioxidant, color
  retention agent)
TBHQ (antioxidant, preservative)

SMOKE POINT	BEST USES	STORAGE IN FRIDGE
495° F.	all-purpose oil up to high-heat cooking (baking, sautéing, frying)	up to 12 months
520° F.	all-purpose oil up to high-heat cooking (baking, sautéing, frying)	up to 12 months
400° F.	all-purpose oil up to medium-high heat cooking (baking/sautéing)	up to 12 months
not applicable	avoid: highly saturated	up to 12 months
320° F.	up to medium-heat cooking (light sautéing, sauces, baking up to 350°F. oven)	up to 4 months
450 F.	up to medium-high heat cooking (baking/sautéing) don't deep-fry: foams & smokes	up to 6 months
not applicable	avoid: usually hydrogenated	not applicable

OILS AT A GLANCE

OIL	PROCESS-ING	PRIMARY FATTY ACID	FLAVOR
flaxseed	unrefined	superunsaturated (57% Omega-3 fatty acids)	nutty/buttery
grapeseed	refined	polyunsaturated	mild
olive	unrefined use extra-virgin, virgin, or "olive oil". Avoid olive pomace oil.	monounsaturated	fruity/nutty
palm/ palm kernel fractionated palm	refined	saturated	mild
peanut	unrefined	monounsaturated	nutty
peanut	refined	monounsaturated	nutty
safflower, reg.	unrefined	polyunsaturated	nutty

SMOKE POINT	BEST USES	STORAGE IN FRIDGE
less than 212 ° F.	no heat/low heat only butter substitute on potatoes, bread, cooked grains. Use in salad dressings, spreads, dips, smoothies	6-8 weeks
400° F.	avoid: only available solvent-extracted	not applicable
350° F.	up to medium-heat cooking (light sautéing, sauces, baking, up to 350 F. oven)	up to 12 months
not applicable	avoid: high in saturated fats	not applicable
320° F.	up to medium-heat cooking (light sautéing, sauces, baking, up to 350° F. oven)	up to 8 months
450° F.	all-purpose oil up to high-heat cooking (baking, sautéing, frying)	up to 12 months
320° F.	up to medium-heat cooking (light sautéing, sauces, baking up to 350° F. oven)	up to 4 months

OILS AT A GLANCE

OIL	PROCESS-ING	PRIMARY FATTY ACID	FLAVOR
safflower, reg.	refined	polyunsaturated	nutty
safflower, high oleic	unrefined	monounsaturated	nutty
	refined	monounsaturated	nutty
sesame	unrefined	monounsaturated/ polyunsaturated	nutty
	refined	monounsaturated/ polyunsaturated	nutty
soy oil	refined	polyunsaturated	bland
sunflower, regular	refined	polyunsaturated	bland
sunflower, high-oleic	unrefined	monounsaturated	nutty
sunflower, high-oleic	refined	monounsaturated	nutty
walnut	refined	polyunsaturated contains 5% Omega 3 fatty acids	slightly nutty

SMOKE POINT	BEST USES	STORAGE IN FRIDGE
450° F.	up to medium-high heat cooking (baking/sautéing) don't deep-fry: high oxidation	up to 6 months
320° F.	up to medium-heat cooking (light sautéing, sauces, baking up to 350° F. oven)	up to 8 months
450° F.	all-purpose oil up to high-heat cooking (baking, sautéing, frying)	up to 12 months
320° F.	up to medium-heat cooking (light sautéing, sauces, baking up to 350° F. oven)	up to 8 months
410° F.	up to medium-high heat cooking (baking, sautéing)	up to 12 months
450° F.	avoid: only available solvent-extracted	not applicable
450° F.	up to medium-high heat cooking (baking, sautéing)	up to 6 months
320° F.	up to medium-heat cooking (light sautéing, sauces, baking up to 350° F. oven)	up to 8 months
450° F.	all-purpose oil up to high-heat cooking (baking, sautéing, frying)	up to 12 months
400° F.	up to medium-high heat cooking (baking, sautéing)	up to 6 months

WORDS TO KNOW ABOUT SWEETENERS AND SWEET FOODS

artificial sweeteners: artificially derived high-intensity sweeteners ranging from 30-600 times the sweetness of table sugar.

Some artificial sweeteners are also calorie-free. Seizures, headaches, mood swings, blurred vision, and other problems have been linked with artificial sweeteners. Although many individuals use artificial sweeteners as a way to cut calories, numerous studies show that those who substitute artificial sweeteners often end up gaining weight rather than losing it as they had hoped. Typically, instead of replacing other sugary, high-fat, high-calorie foods, artificially sweetened foods are often simply added to an already fat-laden diet.

Artifical sweeteners include: acesulfame-K, aspartame, cyclamates, and saccharin.

carob: the dried, roasted, and pulverized pod of the honey locust tree that has a flavor similar to chocolate. It is naturally sweet, very low in fat (unless palm kernel oil or other fats are added), and caffeine-free.

dutch-processed cocoa: cocoa treated with a mild alkali to neutralize the natural acids found in cocoa, modify the flavor, and darken the color.

no added sugars: does not contain any added sweetener or ingredients that contain added sugar. Labeling claim can be used only in products that normally contain added sugars.

organically grown: verified to be grown and produced according to the requirements of the Federal organic certification program using management-intensive methods designed to promote and enhance soil fertility, biological cycles, and biodiversity. No prohibited fertilizers, chemical pesticides, herbicides, or fungicides may have been applied for at least 3 years prior to marketing as organic. Foods labeled as organic are processed, packaged, transported, and stored to retain maximum nutritional value, without the use of artificial preservatives or colorings, irradiation, or toxic synthetic chemicals.

reduced sugar: contains at least 25% less sugar per standard serving size than is typically found in similar products.

refined sugar: sweeteners fully processed to remove naturally occurring fibers and nutrients to concentrate the simple sugars.

sugar-free: contains less than 1/2 gram of sugar per standard serving size.

"unrefined sugar": sweeteners partially processed to remove naturally occurring fibers and nutrients to concentrate the simple sugars.

SWEETS AT A GLANCE

TYPE	SOURCE	USES
amasake	From cooked sweet rice cultured with koji (rice inoculated with Aspergillus orzae) and/or enzymes isolated from sprouted grain.	As beverage or subtle sweetener for breads, pancakes, muffins, cookies, cakes, puddings.
barley malt	From dried sprouted barley mixed with water and cooked until a syrup is produced. Some barley malts are a blend of 60% barley malt and 40% corn malt syrup.	For cookies, muffins, & cakes that can handle a strong flavor.
brown rice syrup	From cooked whole or partially polished brown rice inoculated with sprouted barley or enzymes isolated from sprouted barley to convert the grain's starch into maltose, glucose, and complex carbohydrates. Then cooked into a syrup.	For cakes, muffins, puddings, and sauces: use malted rice syrup. For cookies, candies, sweet spreads, and marinades: use either malted rice syrup or enzyme-treated rice syrup (labeled as brown rice, barley, water, or as cereal enzymes).
corn syrup	From refined corn starch treated with strong acids and enzymes to convert starch to glucose and maltose.	In candies, desserts.

IF REPLACING WHITE SUGAR	STORAGE
Use equal amounts thick amasake, reducing recipe's liquid content by 1/4 cup for each 1 cup of amasake used. Thin amasake beverages may be too diluted to provide much sweetening.	Aseptic-packed: unopened: 6-9 months at room temperature. Opened: 5-7 days in fridge. With refrigerated versions, see dating printed on container.
Use equal amounts to white sugar, reducing the recipe's liquid content by 1/4 cup for each 1 cup barley malt used.	6 months at room temperature or fridge.
Use equal amounts to white sugar, reducing the recipe's liquid content by 1/4 cup for each 1 cup rice syrup used.	6 months at room temperature or fridge.
Use equal amounts to white sugar, reducing the recipe's liquid content by 1/4 cup for each 1 cup corn syrup used.	4-6 months at room temperature.

SWEETS AT A GLANCE

TYPE	SOURCE	USES
date sugar	From dates dried and granulated.	To sweeten breakfast cereals, for streusel & crumb toppings (apply after baking). Can also be combined with hot water to make a syrup.
fructose	From enzyme-treated corn syrup or isolated from refined sugar. Crystalline fructose is 94.5% pure, metabolizing in the body without requiring insulin. High fructose corn syrup metabolizes similarly to sugar.	Beverages, desserts, candies.
fruit juice concentrates	From juice evaporated in a vacuum that retains the fruit's flavor or has the flavor filtered out. Less nutritious versions (available only for manufacturers) may be ultra-clarified to remove all natural colors, flavors, and nutrients from the juice through an ion-exchange process. Thawed frozen fruit juice concentrates can also be used for baking at home.	In beverages, desserts, candies, baked goods.
FruitSource™	From a blend of grape juice concentrate and brown rice syrup. Available both granular and liquid.	In desserts, baked goods.

IF REPLACING WHITE SUGAR

STORAGE

Use 2/3-1 cup to substitute for 1 cup white sugar. If substituting for a liquid sweetener, increase the recipe's dry ingredients by 1/3 cup for every 2/3 cup date sugar used.

12 months at room temperature.

Only crystalline or liquid fructose from crystalline fructose is available for home use. Use 1/2-2/3 cup to substitute for 1 cup white sugar. For best results, use recipes specially formulated for sweetening with fructose.

12 months at room temperature.

If using thawed frozen juice concentrate: use equal amounts to white sugar, reducing the recipe's liquid content by 1/4 cup for every 1 cup concentrate used. When baking, add 1/4-1/2 tsp. baking soda for each 1 cup concentrate used. If using thick fruit juice concentrate sold in a jar, use 1/2-2/3 cup to replace 1 cup white sugar, reducing recipe's liquid content and adding baking soda as outlined above.

8-12 months freezer 7-10 days fridge.

Granular: Use equal amounts to white sugar. Liquid: Use equal amounts to white sugar, reducing the recipe's liquid content by 1/4 cup per 1 cup liquid FruitSource™ used

6 months at room temperature.

SWEETS AT A GLANCE

TYPE	SOURCE	USES
honey	From flower nectar converted by bees into a sweetener. Once removed from the hive, the honey is heated to extract it from the comb and then strained, sometimes also filtered. **Never give raw honey to children under the age of 1 year. Raw honey may harbor spores of clostridium botulinum which can germinate and grow in infants whose immune systems are still under-developed. Symptoms may include lethargy and difficulty feeding, leading possibly to death if left unchecked.	In desserts, baked goods, marinades, sauces, spreads.
jams/ jellies	From fruit and/or fruit juice cooked with sugar or fruit juice concentrates.	In spreads, fillings.
maple syrup	From maple tree sap cooked and concentrated.	In desserts, baked goods, toppings.

IF REPLACING WHITE SUGAR

Use 1/2-2/3 cup honey to replace 1 cup white sugar, reducing the recipe's liquid content by 1/4 cup for each 1 cup honey used. In baked goods, add 1/4 tsp. baking soda per 1 cup honey to neutralize its acidity.

STORAGE

12 months at room temperature.

Not applicable.

Unopened: 1 year at room temperature. Opened: 6 months in fridge.

Use 1/2-2/3 cup to replace 1 cup white sugar, reducing the recipe's liquid content by 1/4 cup.

Up to 12 months in fridge.

SWEETS AT A GLANCE

TYPE	SOURCE	USES
molasses	*Blackstrap:* final syrup left from crystallizing the sucrose from sugar cane. *Barbados:* made by slowly boiling filtered sugar cane juice into a syrup. *Sorghum:* the concentrated juice from the sweet sorghum plant.	In desserts and baked goods that can handle a strong flavor.
refined sugars: brown & white	From sugar cane or sugar beet juice concentrated and granulated, fully refined to remove molasses, and all accompanying nutrients. Brown sugar is white sugar sprayed with molasses.	In desserts, baked goods, candies, toppings.
"unrefined sugars": demarara, evaporated cane juice, muscovado, turbinado	From sugar cane or sugar beet juice concentrated and granulated, preserving the naturally occurring molasses. *Demarara:* coarsely ground, large, slightly sticky, golden crystals. *Evaporated cane juice:* finely ground, light brown crystals. *Muscovado:* molasses boiled down and crystallized, slightly coarse and sticky. *Turbinado:* moderately fine, golden brown crystals.	In desserts, baked goods, candies.

IF REPLACING WHITE SUGAR

Use equal amounts to white sugar, reducing the recipe's liquid content by 1/4 cup for each cup molasses used.

STORAGE

12-24 months at room temperature.

Not applicable.

Indefinitely at room temperature.

Use equal amounts to white sugar.

Indefinitely at room temperature.

JELLY/ JAMS/ SYRUP ADDITIVES TO AVOID

artificial color

artificial flavor

potassium sorbate (preservative, antimycotic agent)

sodium benzoate (preservative, antimycotic agent)

sorbic acid (preservative, antimycotic agent)

sulfur dioxide (preservative, antioxidant, color retention agent)

CANDY/CONFECTIONS ADDITIVES TO AVOID

artificial color

artificial flavor

artificial sweeteners

caprenin (fat substitute)

hydrogenated fats (treated to prolong shelf life and to provide texture and body)

partially hydrogenated fats (treated to prolong shelf life and to provide texture and body)

sodium benzoate (preservative, antimycotic agent)

sulfur dioxide (preservative, antioxidant, color retention agent)

TBHQ (antioxidant, preservative)

vanillin (artificial flavor)

COOKIES/DESSERT ADDITIVES TO AVOID

artificial color

artificial flavor

bleached flour (artificially aged flour)

partially hydrogenated oil (treated to prolong shelf life and to provide texture and body)

potassium sorbate (preservative, antimycotic agent)

sodium benzoate (preservative, antimycotic agent)

sulfur dioxide (preservative, antioxidant, color retention agent)

vanillin (artificial flavor)

SWEET DRINK ADDITIVES TO AVOID

artificial flavor

artificial sweeteners

brominated vegetable oil (flavor carrier)

calcium disodium EDTA (antioxidant, sequestrant)

potassium benzoate (preservative, antimycotic agent)

sodium benzoate (preservative, antimycotic agent)

THE QUICK MEAL PANTRY

Even though time often seems to be at a premium, there's no need to put nutrition on the back burner. Just keep a variety of the following quick-cooking foods on hand to make delicious *Good Food* meals in 30 minutes or less.

GRAINS
basmati rice
buckwheat
bulgur
couscous
millet
mochi
pancake/biscuit mixes
pastas (stock a variety of shapes, sizes, flavors)
pilaf mixes
ramen
quinoa
seitan (wheat meat)
texmati™ rice

BREADS
chapatis
crackers
crusty sourdough breads
focaccia
naan
pita bread
pizza crust
rice cakes
tortillas

VEGETABLES
Always have fresh veggies around. The following varieties have longer storage life.

broccoli
cabbage
canned tomato products
carrots and other root
veggies
frozen peas, etc.
garlic
mushrooms, dried

salad greens medley
  (available prewashed in
  packages)
onion

parsley
potatoes
sauerkraut
tomatoes, dried

FRUIT
apples
dried fruits (raisins, etc.)

lemons
oranges

MEATS
ground beef/round
sirloin tip, etc. cut in stir-fry strips

POULTRY
chicken tenderloin strips
ground chicken/turkey

skinned & boned chicken breasts
eggs

FISH
canned tuna, salmon,
sardines

fresh/frozen fish fillets and steaks
frozen fish medallions

BEANS
canned soups
dry miso soup mix
falafel mix
frozen tofu or tempeh
burgers
green lentils

instant hummus mix
precooked canned beans
prepared bean dips
red lentils
tempeh
tofu

NUTS
Great for garnishing entrées and snacks

almond butter
almonds
peanut butter

peanuts
pecans
pinenuts

sesame tahini
sunflower seeds

DAIRY (milk- or soy-based)
cheese (misc. varieties)
Parmesan cheese
yogurt

CONDIMENTS
balsamic vinegar
brown rice vinegar
chile peppers
mustards
olive oil
olive pastes
olives
pasta sauces
pesto

salad dressings
salsas
sesame oil
tamari/tamari shoyu (soy
  sauce)
umeboshi plums/paste
umeboshi vinegar
wine vinegars

QUICK MEAL PLANNING HINTS

1. Keep it simple: center the meal around one item and fill in the accompaniments.

2. Plan in technicolor: meals that are eye-appealing will be more satisfying.

3. Think textures: variety in textures (soft, crunchy, slightly firm, creamy) will make meals more satisfying.

4. Serve it in style: simple garnishing and attention to presentation can make a quick meal look special. Invest in a few colorful platters and bowls. Top entrées with chopped green onions, a sprig of fresh herbs, chopped nuts, or a tablespoon of grated carrot or beet.

CONVENIENCE FOOD ADDITIVES TO AVOID

CANNED SOUP
disodium guanylate (flavor enhancer)
disodium inosinate (flavor enhancer)
monosodium glutamate (MSG) (flavor enhancer)
partially hydrogenated oil (treated to prolong shelf
    life and to provide texture and body)

BOUILLON/SOUP MIX
artificial color
BHA (antioxidant, preservative)
BHT (antioxidant, preservative)
monosodium glutamate (MSG) (antioxidant,
    preservative)
sodium bisulfite (preservative, antioxidant, color
    retention agent)
sodium sulfite (preservative, antioxidant, color
    retention agent)
sulfur dioxide (preservative, antioxidant, color
    retention agent)

CHIPS/SNACKS
artificial color
artificial flavor
disodium guanylate (flavor enhancer)
disodium inosinate (flavor enhancer)
monosodium glutamate (MSG) (flavor enhancer)
partially hydrogenated oil (treated to prolong shelf

life and to provide texture and body)
TBHQ (antioxidant, preservative)

FROZEN DINNERS
artificial flavor
BHT (antioxidant, preservative)
calcium disodium EDTA (antioxidant, sequestrant)
calcium propionate (antimycotic agent)
disodium guanylate (flavor enhancer)
disodium inosinate (flavor enhancer)
monosodium glutamate (MSG) (flavor enhancer)
partially hydrogenated oil (treated to prolong shelf
   life and to provide texture and body)
potassium sorbate (preservative, antimycotic agent)
sodium nitrite (antioxidant, flavor, color retention
   agent)

QUICK DINNER MIXES
artificial color
artificial flavor
disodium guanylate (flavor enhancer)
disodium inosinate (flavor enhancer)
monosodium glutamate (MSG) (flavor enhancer)
partially hydrogenated oil (treated to prolong shelf
   life and to provide texture and body)
sodium bisulfite (preservative, antioxidant, color
   retention agent)
sodium sulfite (preservative, antioxidant, color
   retention agent)

SAUCES/MARINADES
artificial color
artificial flavor
potassium sorbate (preservative, antimycotic agent)
sodium benzoate (preservative, antimycotic agent)

FROZEN DESSERTS
artificial color
artificial flavor
calcium disodium EDTA (antioxidant, sequestrant)
partially hydrogenated oil (treated to prolong shelf
   life and to provide texture and body)
sodium benzoate (preservative, antimycotic agent)
sodium stearoyl-2-lactylate (emulsifier, whipping
   agent)

WORDS TO KNOW ABOUT SEASONINGS/ CONDIMENTS

apple cider vinegar: a tart, apple-flavored vinegar produced from hard apple cider. Use in salad dressings and as a general condiment.

balsamic vinegar: a dark, dense, syrupy vinegar that is both sweet and slightly tart—the result of a complex aging process that involves transferring the vinegar each year into increasingly smaller barrels. Use in salad dressings, marinades, and as a condiment for fruit, vegetables, and grains.

fruit vinegar: light, fresh-flavored vinegar made by infusing the flavor of raspberry, strawberry, or blueberry into white wine vinegar. Use in salad dressings, marinades, and as a condiment on vegetables, fruit salads, and grains.

gomasio (also known as sesame salt): a low-sodium alternative to salt made from ground roasted sesame seeds and sea salt. Use as a condiment on cooked vegetables, grains, and beans.

herbs: the leaves of low-growing annual or perennial plants that are usually grown in temperate climates.

herb vinegar: cider, red wine, or white wine vinegars steeped with herbs. Use on salads.

kosher salt: salt that has larger crystals, claimed to give foods a brighter taste than typical table salt.

malt vinegar: a distinctly flavored vinegar made by fermenting the liquid extract of malted barley. Use in hot and cold vegetable dishes, sautéed potatoes, and, of course, fish and chips.

mirin: a sweet cooking wine made from sweet rice, rice koji, and water. (Avoid those that contain sugar and chemical fermenting agents.) Use in marinades, salad dressings, sauces, noodle dishes, vegetables, and in overly pungent or salty dishes that need rebalancing.

miso: a fermented soybean paste made by mixing cooked soybeans or chickpeas with koji (grain inoculated with Aspergillus orzae), salt, water, and, in some varieties, grain. Depending on the type of miso, the mixture is then fermented from 2 months to 3 years. Use in soups or sauces instead of bouillon or as a base for stews, gravies, salad dressings, dips, or spreads.

mustard: a condiment whose flavors vary according to the type of mustard seed, texture, whether it includes wine or vinegar, and the particular types of herbs and spices used. Yellow mustard seeds are mild, brown are pungent, and oriental are sharp in flavor. Most mustards are made from a combination of seeds rather than one variety.

pickled ginger: a condiment made from young, tender, thinly sliced ginger roots that are briefly salt pressed and pickled in rice vinegar and shiso leaves. (Avoid varieties made with preservatives and artificial color.) Serve with sushi, nori maki, and other entrées for flavor and color. It's also delicious as an addition to sandwiches and dips.

rice vinegar (also known as rice wine vinegar): a slightly sweet, smooth, mellow flavor with about half the sharpness of cider vinegar. Brown rice vinegar has a more full-bodied taste than white rice vinegar. Use in salad dressings, sauces, and as a condiment on fish, vegetables, and grain dishes.

sea salt: salt extracted from salt water. In addition to sodium chloride, unrefined sea salt retains many of the trace minerals originally found in the sea. Refined sea salt contains few, if any, trace minerals. Neither contains naturally occurring iodine. Both should be used in moderation.

seeds: the seeds of various annual plants used for seasoning.

sherry vinegar: a mellow, full-bodied flavor with a sweet aftertaste. Use in dressings for fruit salads and vegetable salads featuring cheeses.

shiso leaf powder: a salty/sour condiment made from the dried purple leaves of the beefsteak plant which are pickled with umeboshi plums. Use on vegetables, salads, or grains.

shoyu (also known as "tamari shoyu"): naturally produced soy sauce made from soybeans, wheat, water, and sea salt. It has a rich, savory aroma and a sweeter flavor than tamari. It is best added at the end of cooking or as a condiment.

spices: dried tropical grown barks, roots, or fruits/berries from perennial shrubs.

table salt: highly refined salt mined from salt mines or from salt water. It often contains iodine and additives to make it free-flowing. Compared to sea salt and kosher salt, its flavor is fairly mediocre.

tamari: naturally produced, wheat-free soy sauce made from soybeans, water, and sea salt. It has a stronger, deeper flavor than shoyu and is best added to foods while they are cooking.

umeboshi plum: sour, green Japanese plums that are pickled with sea salt and shiso, the purple leaves from the beefsteak plant. Use to impart a sour/salty flavor in dips, spreads, sauces, grains, and broths.

umeboshi vinegar: a salty, tart-flavored condiment that is not a true vinegar but the liquid drawn off from pickled umeboshi plums and shiso leaves. Use in salad dressings, dips, marinades, and as a condiment on vegetables, beans, and grains.

wasabi: Japanese powdered horseradish that is less sharp and more aromatic than regular horseradish. High quality wasabi has a dull, greenish color; avoid artificially colored varieties. Mix equal amounts of water and wasabi to form a paste. Cover and let sit for 10 minutes to mingle flavors.

wine vinegar: made from either red or white wines. Red wine vinegar is more pungent and best with strong-flavored greens, meats, cheese dishes, and salads. White wine vinegar has a more delicate flavor and is best with mild-tasting greens.

SODIUM EQUIVALENCY CHART
1/2 teaspoon

mustard:	33 mg.
gomasio :	40 mg.
white miso:	68 mg.
olive (1 large ripe):	120 mg.
brown rice miso:	135 mg.
tamari:	157 mg.
ume plum paste:	235 mg.
olives (3 green):	280 mg.
pickles (4 dill):	310 mg.
salt:	1150 mg.

COOKING STAPLES STORAGE GUIDELINES

TYPE	ROOM TEMP.	REFRIGERATOR
baking powder	6 months	N/A
baking soda	18 months	N/A
baking yeast (dry & fresh)	N/A	to dating on label
cornstarch	12 months	N/A
flavor extracts	3-4 months*	N/A
herbs/spices		
dried ground	6 months	N/A
dried whole	12 months	N/A
fresh	N/A	1 week**
hot sauce	12 months (unopened)	6 months (opened)
ketchup	12 months (unopened)	6 months (opened)
mayonnaise	12 months (unopened)	6 months (opened)
mustard	12 months (unopened)	6 months (opened)
tabasco	12 months	N/A
salad dressings	12 months (unopened)	6 months (opened)
salt	indefinitely	N/A
tamari/soy sauce	12 months	N/A
vinegars	12 months	N/A

N/A: not applicable.
*Won't spoil but flavor starts to diminish.
**Place stems in water, cover with plastic bag.

SEASONINGS/SEASONING MIXES ADDITIVES TO AVOID

artificial color
artificial flavor
BHA (antioxidant, preservative)
monosodium glutamate (MSG) (flavor enhancer)
partially hydrogenated oil (treated to prolong shelf
  life and to provide texture and body)
sulfiting agents (preservative, antioxidant, color
  retention agent)
sulfur dioxide (preservative, antioxidant, color
  retention agent)

CONDIMENTS/SAUCES ADDITIVES TO AVOID

artificial color
calcium disodium EDTA (antioxidant, sequestrant)
disodium guanylate (flavor enhancer)
disodium inosinate (flavor enhancer)
potassium sorbate (preservative, antimycotic agent)
sodium benzoate (preservative, antimycotic agent)

U.S. WEIGHTS AND MEASURES

teaspoons/tablespoons

pinch/dash	less than 1/8 teaspoon
3 teaspoons	1 tablespoon
1/2 tablespoon	1 1/2 teaspoon
1 tablespoon	1/2 fluid ounce
4 tablespoons	1/4 cup or 2 fluid ounces
5 1/3 tablespoons	1/3 cup or 3 fluid ounces
8 tablespoons	1/2 cup or 4 fluid ounces
12 tablespoons	3/4 cup or 6 fluid ounces
16 tablespoons	1 cup or 8 fluid ounces

cups/pints/quarts/gallons

1 cup	1/2 pint or 8 fluid ounces
2 cups	1 pint or 16 fluid ounces
4 cups	1 quart or 32 fluid ounces
2 quarts	1/2 gallon
4 quarts	1 gallon

ounces/pounds

2 ounces	1/8 pound
4 ounces	1/4 pound
5 1/3 ounces	1/3 pound
8 ounces	1/2 pound
10 2/3 ounces	2/3 pound
12 ounces	3/4 pound
16 ounces	1 pound

METRIC WEIGHTS/MEASURES

milliliters/liters

4.9 milliliters	1 teaspoon
14.8 milliliters	1 tablespoon
236.6 milliliters	1 cup
946.4 milliliters	1 quart
1 deciliter	6 2/3 tablespoons
1/4 liter	1 cup + 2 1/4 teaspoons
1/2 liter	1 pint + 4 1/2 teaspoons
1 liter	1000 milliliters or 1.06 quarts (1 quart + scant 1/4 cup)

grams/kilograms

1 gram	0.0353 ounces
28.35 grams	1 ounce
100 grams	3 1/2 ounces
227 grams	8 ounces or 1/2 pound
453.59 grams	16 ounces or 1 pound
1000 grams	1 kilogram
1 kilogram	2.21 pounds or 2 pounds 3 1/4 ounces

METRIC CONVERSION FACTORS

ounces to grams	multiply ounces by 28.35
grams to ounces	multiply grams by 0.353
pounds to grams	multiply pounds by 453. 59
ounces to milliliters	multiply ounces by 30
cups to liters	multiply cups by 0.24

154

NOTES

NOTES

**The Crossing Press publishes a full
selection of titles on
cooking and health.
To receive our current catalog,
please call toll-free, 800-777-1048.**